THE VEGGIE BIBLE: EVERY TYPE OF VEGGIE FOR YOUR BENEFIT

TELESHA CUTLER

AUTHOR NOTE

For those who are on the journey to better wellness and health, nutrition is if not the most important factor in that besides mental and spiritual aspects. As my students have followed my articles and post I have compiled a collection of those which help teach people about veggies and their benefits. Therefore buckle up and let's take this journey together.

CONTENTS

The Power of Spinach: Discover the Incredible Health Benefits of Eating Spinach 4

Kale: The Superfood You Need for a Healthier Lifestyle................................6

Carrots: The Crunchy Superfood That Will Keep You Healthy and Happy! 8

The Amazing Benefits of Eating Broccoli and How it Can Boost Your Health................................10

The Incredible Health Benefits of Eating Garlic Regularly: What Science Says.................................12

Why Brussel Sprouts Should Be Your New Favorite Vegetable: The Surprising Health Benefits. 14

The Incredible Health Benefits of Eating Swiss Chard: What You Need to Know! 16

The Amazing Benefits of Eating Beets: Why You Should Add Beets to Your Diet.................................18

The Many Benefits of Eating Asparagus: Why You Should Add It to Your Diet.................................20

The Incredible Health Benefits of Eating Red Cabbage You Need to Know!................................22

Fire Up Your Health: Discovering the Benefits of Eating Jalapeno Pepper. 24

Mushroom Power: Exploring the Health Benefits of Adding Mushrooms to Your Diet.....................26

The Amazing Health Benefits of Adding Butternut Squash to Your Diet. 28

From Jack-O-Lanterns to Superfoods: The Surprising Health Benefits of Pumpkin.....................30

The Surprising Health Benefits of Eating Red Bell Peppers.................................32

Radicchio: The Superfood You Should Be Eating Today! 34

Incredible Health Benefits of Adding Endive to Your Diet.................................36

The Power of Cauliflower: Surprising Health Benefits You Need to Know. 38

Discover the Amazing Benefits of Eating Kohlrabi: The Superfood You Need in Your Diet................40

The Incredible Health Benefits of Watercress You Need to Know About! 42

The Incredible Health Benefits of Eating Turnip Greens You Need to Know.................................44

Why Bok Choy is the Ultimate Superfood You Need to Add to Your Diet! 46

"Napa Cabbage: The Nutrient-Packed Superfood You Need in Your Diet" 48

The Incredible Benefits of Adding Arugula to Your Diet: A Comprehensive Guide. 50

Why Green Leaf Lettuce is the Ultimate Superfood for Your Health. 52

Chicory Greens: The Nutritious and Delicious Addition to Your Diet.................................54

Radish: A Crunchy and Nutritious Delight! Exploring the Health Benefits of Eating Radish.................56

Here Are The Incredible Health Benefits of Eating Basil Every Day. 58

The Secret Benefits of Cilantro: Why You Should Add it to Your Diet Today.................................60

The Power of Parsley: Surprising Health Benefits You Need to Know! 62

The Power of Spinach: Discover the Incredible Health Benefits of Eating Spinach

When it comes to healthy eating, spinach is one of the most nutrient-dense foods available. Packed with vitamins and minerals, this leafy green has been known to have plenty of health benefits for decades. Not only is spinach low in calories, but it can also help improve your eyesight, strengthen your bones, improve your cardiovascular health and even help with reducing the risk of cancer. Spinach can be eaten raw, cooked, or blended as part of a smoothie, making it a versatile and easy-to-use ingredient to add to your diet. In this article, we will explore the power of spinach and the incredible health benefits of including this superfood in your daily diet.

1. What is spinach?
Spinach is a leafy green vegetable that is packed with nutrition. It's part of the Amaranthaceae family and is related to beets and quinoa. The plant has dark green leaves that are flat and slightly crinkled, with a slightly bitter taste. Spinach is a versatile vegetable that can be eaten raw in salads or cooked in a variety of dishes. It can be boiled, steamed, sautéed, or roasted. Spinach is rich in vitamins and minerals, including vitamin A, vitamin C, vitamin K, folate, iron, and calcium. It is also a great source of protein and fiber. Eating spinach regularly can help to lower blood pressure, prevent cancer, and improve bone health. It is also known to be good for your eyesight, your skin, and your immune system. Spinach is a healthy addition to any diet, and it's easy to incorporate into your meals. Whether you choose to eat it raw or cooked, spinach is a nutritious and delicious vegetable that can help you to feel your best.

2. Nutritional value of spinach
Spinach is a superfood packed with essential nutrients that can benefit your overall health. It is a rich source of vitamins A, C, K, and folic acid. It also contains essential minerals such as iron, calcium, and potassium. Spinach is low in calories and has a high water content, making it an excellent choice for weight loss diets. Moreover, it is a great source of dietary fiber, which can help to improve digestion and reduce constipation. Spinach is also rich in antioxidants, which can help to reduce the risk of chronic diseases such as cancer, heart disease, and diabetes. The vitamins and minerals found in spinach can also help to support healthy bones, teeth, and skin. Additionally, spinach is an excellent source of plant-based protein, making it a great choice for vegetarians and vegans. Overall, spinach is a nutrient-dense food that can provide numerous health benefits when included in a balanced diet.

3. Health benefits of spinach
Spinach is a leafy green vegetable packed with a variety of health benefits. The nutrients found in spinach can benefit almost every part of your body. For starters, spinach is high in vitamins A and C, which are both powerful antioxidants. These antioxidants help to protect your cells from damage caused by free radicals. Spinach is also high in fiber, which can help keep your digestive system healthy and prevent constipation. Additionally, spinach is a good source of iron, which is essential for the production of red blood cells. This makes it an important food for people who suffer from anemia. Spinach also contains magnesium and potassium, which are important minerals that help to regulate blood pressure. Furthermore, spinach is low in calories and high in water content, making it an excellent food choice for those looking to lose weight. The health benefits of spinach are numerous, and it's a great addition to any diet. Whether you're looking to improve your overall health or just want to add some extra nutrition to your meals, spinach is defiitely a superfood that you should consider incorporating into your diet.

4. How to incorporate spinach into your diet

Spinach is a powerhouse of nutrients and has a ton of health benefits. If you're looking for ways to incorporate spinach into your diet, there are many easy and delicious ways to do it. One of the best ways to enjoy spinach is in a salad. Simply toss a handful of spinach leaves with some cherry tomatoes, cucumber, and feta cheese for a refreshing and healthy meal. You can also add spinach to smoothies for a boost of nutrients. Just blend together some spinach, banana, and almond milk for a healthy and delicious breakfast. Spinach is also fantastic in omelets. Just mix some spinach with eggs and cheese for a quick and easy meal. Finally, you can add spinach to your pasta dishes. Simply sauté some spinach with garlic and olive oil and add it to your favorite pasta dish. The possibilities are endless when it comes to incorporating spinach into your diet. Not only is spinach delicious, but it's also incredibly good for you. So why not give it a try?

Kale: The Superfood You Need for a Healthier Lifestyle.

As we get older, we start to realize that the old adage "you are what you eat" has a lot of truth to it. We all want to live healthy lives and feel our best, but with so much conflicting information out there about what foods are good for us, it can be overwhelming to know where to start. That's where kale comes in. This leafy green vegetable is packed with essential vitamins and minerals that can help keep your body healthy and functioning at its best. Not only is kale a superfood, but it's also delicious and versatile, making it easy to incorporate into your daily meals. So if you're looking to take your health to the next level, keep reading to find out why kale should be a staple in your diet.

1. What is kale and why is it considered a superfood?
Kale is a leafy green vegetable that has gained popularity in recent years for its many health benefits. It is considered a superfood because it is packed with vitamins, minerals, and antioxidants that are essential for maintaining good health. Kale is a great source of vitamin C, vitamin K, vitamin A, and vitamin B6. It is also high in fiber, calcium, potassium, and iron. One of the most significant benefits of kale is its high level of antioxidants, which help to protect the body from harmful free radicals. These antioxidants may also help to reduce the risk of chronic diseases such as heart disease, cancer, and diabetes. In addition to its health benefits, kale is also a versatile vegetable that can be used in a variety of dishes. It can be eaten raw in salads, sautéed as a side dish, or blended into smoothies. With its many benefits and versatility, kale is definitely a superfood that everyone should consider incorporating into their diet.

2. The nutritional benefits of kale
Kale is one of the most nutrient-dense foods on the planet, and it has quickly gained a reputation as a superfood. The nutritional benefits of kale are truly impressive. It is an excellent source of vitamins A, C, and K, as well as calcium, iron, and antioxidants. One cup of kale contains only 33 calories, but it also contains three grams of protein and two grams of fiber. This combination of nutrients makes kale an excellent choice for anyone who is looking to improve their health. The vitamin A in kale is beneficial for eye health, while the vitamin C helps to boost the immune system. The vitamin K helps with blood clotting, and the calcium helps to build strong bones. The iron in kale helps to build red blood cells, which can improve energy levels. Additionally, the antioxidants in kale help to protect the body against damage from free radicals. Overall, including kale in your diet can have a significant impact on your health and well-being.

3. How to incorporate kale into your diet
Kale is a nutrient-dense superfood that is packed with vitamins and minerals. It has become increasingly popular in recent years, and for good reason. But how do you incorporate kale into your diet? Here are a few simple ways to add kale to your meals: 1. Add kale to your salads. Kale is a great addition to any salad. Simply chop up the kale and mix it in with your other greens. You can also add some nuts or seeds for extra crunch. 2. Make a kale smoothie. Kale is perfect for smoothies. Just blend some kale with your favorite fruits and a bit of yogurt or milk for a delicious and nutritious drink. 3. Use kale in your soups and stews. Kale can add a lot of flavor to your favorite soups and stews. Simply chop up some kale and add it to your pot. 4. Sautee kale with some garlic and olive oil. This is a quick and easy way to add some extra greens to your meal. Sautee the kale with some garlic and olive oil until it is tender. Incorporating kale into your diet is easy and beneficial for your health. Whether you choose to add it to your salads, smoothies, soups, or sautee it with some garlic and olive oil, kale is a versatile and nutritious superfood that you will definitely want to incorporate into your meals.

4. Conclusion.
In conclusion, kale is undoubtedly one of the healthiest vegetables you can eat. Its numerous benefits make it a true superfood that can have a significant positive impact on your health and well-being. Adding kale to your diet is an excellent way to boost your immune system, reduce inflammation, and improve your overall health. It's easy to add kale to your diet, whether you prefer to eat it raw in salads, sautéed as a side dish, or blended into smoothies. So, if you're looking for a simple way to improve your health and wellness, incorporating kale into your diet is an excellent place to start. Start small, and gradually add it to your meals to discover the many benefits it has to offer.

Carrots: The Crunchy Superfood That Will Keep You Healthy and Happy!

When you think of healthy eating, the humble carrot may not be the first food that comes to mind. However, this crunchy superfood is packed with nutrients that can help keep you healthy and happy. Carrots contain high levels of beta-carotene, an antioxidant that helps with immune function and protects your skin from sun damage. They are also rich in vitamin A, which is essential for maintaining healthy vision, and vitamin K, which helps with blood clotting. Additionally, carrots are a great source of fiber, which aids in digestion and helps you feel full. In this article, we'll delve deeper into the benefits of carrots and explore creative ways to incorporate this versatile vegetable into your diet. Get ready to add this crunchy superfood to your grocery list!

1. The nutritional benefits of carrots

Carrots are a crunchy superfood that is not only tasty but also incredibly nutritious. They are low in calories, high in fiber, and packed with essential vitamins and minerals. One of the main nutrients that carrots are known for is beta-carotene, which is converted to vitamin A in the body. Vitamin A is essential for healthy vision, immune system function, and skin health. Carrots are also a good source of vitamin K, which is important for blood clotting and bone health. Additionally, they contain antioxidants such as lutein and zeaxanthin, which may help to reduce the risk of chronic diseases such as cancer and heart disease. Carrots are also rich in potassium, which is important for maintaining healthy blood pressure levels. They are also a good source of vitamin C, which is needed for collagen production and helps to support healthy skin and joints. Finally, carrots are packed with fiber, which can help to promote healthy digestion and keep you feeling full for longer. As you can see, there are many nutritional benefits to eating carrots, making them an excellent addition to any healthy diet.

2. How to incorporate carrots into your diet

Carrots are a delicious and healthy vegetable that can be easily incorporated into your diet. There are many different ways to enjoy carrots, whether raw, cooked, or blended into a smoothie. One simple way to incorporate carrots into your diet is to simply snack on them. Carrots are crunchy and make the perfect snack to munch on throughout the day. You can also add them to a salad for a flavorful and nutritious addition. Another way to enjoy carrots is to roast them in the oven. Simply cut them into sticks, season with your favorite herbs and spices, and roast until tender. Roasted carrots make a delicious side dish and are a great alternative to other starchy vegetables. For those who love to cook, carrots can be used in a variety of recipes. From soups to stews, to casseroles, carrots add a sweet and savory flavor to any dish. Lastly, for those who are looking for a quick and easy way to incorporate carrots into their diet, consider blending them into a smoothie. Carrot smoothies are a great way to start your day and provide a boost of energy and nutrients. With so many delicious and healthy ways to enjoy carrots, there is no excuse not to incorporate them into your diet.

3. Creative recipes using carrots

Carrots are a versatile and healthy vegetable that can be used in a variety of dishes. Here are some creative recipes that highlight the delicious, crunchy goodness of carrots: 1. Carrot hummus: Combine cooked carrots with chickpeas, tahini, lemon juice, and garlic in a food processor and blend until smooth. Serve with pita bread or vegetables. 2. Carrot fries: Cut carrots into long, thin strips, toss with olive oil and seasonings, and bake in the oven until crispy. Serve with a dipping sauce of your choice. 3. Carrot cake pancakes: Mix grated carrots, cinnamon, nutmeg, and vanilla into pancake batter and cook as usual. Top with cream cheese frosting and chopped nuts. 4. Carrot and quinoa salad: Cook quinoa according to package instructions and mix with grated carrots, chopped herbs, nuts, and a vinaigrette dressing. 5. Carrot soup: Cook chopped carrots with onions, garlic, and broth until tender, then blend until smooth. Add cream or coconut milk for a creamy texture. These creative recipes not only showcase the delicious and nutritious carrot but also make healthy eating fun and exciting.

4. Conclusion.

In conclusion, carrots are a delicious and crunchy superfood that provides numerous health benefits. They are packed with vitamins, minerals, and antioxidants that can help keep you healthy and happy. Whether you eat them raw, roasted, or cooked, carrots are a versatile and tasty addition to any meal. Not only do they help maintain healthy eyesight and skin, but they also boost the immune system and promote healthy digestion. With so many health benefits, there is no reason not to add carrots to your diet. So go ahead and enjoy this nutritious and delicious crunchy superfood!

The Amazing Benefits of Eating Broccoli and How it Can Boost Your Health

Broccoli is often considered one of the healthiest vegetables on the planet. It's packed with vitamins, minerals, and antioxidants that have a positive impact on your overall health. Despite its many benefits, broccoli is often overlooked or avoided because of its taste, texture, or smell. However, it's worth giving broccoli a chance as it can enhance your health and well-being in more ways than you might think. In this article, we'll explore the amazing benefits that broccoli has to offer and how it can boost your health. From aiding digestion and reducing inflammation to supporting a healthy immune system and even preventing cancer, you'll be amazed at what this cruciferous vegetable can do for your body. So, let's dive in and discover how broccoli can transform your health!

1. What is broccoli and its nutritional value?
Broccoli is a cruciferous vegetable that is packed with nutrients and health benefits. It is closely related to other vegetables like kale, cauliflower, and Brussels sprouts. Broccoli is low in calories and high in fiber, making it a great choice for those who are looking to maintain a healthy diet. When it comes to nutritional value, broccoli is rich in vitamin C, vitamin K, vitamin A, and folate. It also contains small amounts of other important minerals like calcium, iron, and potassium. Additionally, broccoli is a great source of antioxidants, which can help to reduce inflammation in the body and protect against chronic diseases like cancer, diabetes, and heart disease. Eating broccoli regularly can also help to boost your immune system, maintain healthy skin, and aid in digestion. With all of these amazing nutritional benefits, it's no wonder why broccoli is considered a superfood!

2. How broccoli can aid digestion and reduce inflammation
Broccoli is a superfood that is packed with nutrients that can help your body in many ways. One of the ways that broccoli can aid your health is by improving your digestion system. Broccoli is a great source of fiber, which is essential for good digestion. Fiber can help to keep your digestive system working smoothly and can prevent constipation. In addition, broccoli contains a unique compound called sulforaphane, which has been shown to reduce inflammation in the digestive tract. This can be particularly helpful for people who suffer from inflammatory bowel diseases such as Crohn's disease or ulcerative colitis. Inflammation is a natural response to injury or infection, but chronic inflammation can be harmful to the body. By consuming broccoli regularly, you can reduce inflammation in your digestive tract and improve your overall digestive health. So, if you are looking for an easy and delicious way to improve your digestion, try adding more broccoli to your diet.

3. How broccoli can support a healthy immune system and prevent cancer
Broccoli is a superfood that has been shown to have incredible health benefits. One of the most significant benefits of eating broccoli is that it can help support a healthy immune system. Broccoli is rich in vitamin C, which is essential for a strong immune system. Vitamin C helps to stimulate the production of white blood cells, which are responsible for fighting off infections and diseases. Additionally, broccoli contains antioxidants that help to protect the immune system from damage caused by free radicals. Another amazing benefit of eating broccoli is its potential to prevent cancer. Broccoli contains compounds called sulforaphane and isothiocyanates, which have been shown to have anti-cancer properties. These compounds work by reducing inflammation in the body, which is a significant risk factor for cancer. They also help to inhibit the growth of cancer cells and can even cause them to self-destruct. Studies have

shown that people who eat broccoli regularly have a lower risk of developing certain cancers, such as breast, prostate, and lung cancer. Additionally, eating broccoli has also been shown to reduce the risk of other chronic diseases, such as heart disease and diabetes. Incorporating broccoli into your diet is an easy way to boost your health and support your immune system. Whether you enjoy it raw in a salad or steamed as a side dish, broccoli is a delicious and nutritious addition to any meal.

4. How to incorporate broccoli into your diet
Broccoli is a powerhouse of essential vitamins and minerals that can help boost your overall health. It is a versatile vegetable that can be incorporated into your diet in a variety of ways. Here are some tips on how to incorporate broccoli into your diet: 1. Add broccoli to your salads: Add some chopped broccoli to your salad to give it a healthy crunch and boost of nutrients. 2. Make a broccoli soup: Broccoli soup is easy to make, delicious, and nutritious. You can make it creamy or chunky, depending on your preference. 3. Use broccoli in your stir-fry: Broccoli is a great addition to any stir-fry. Simply add some broccoli florets to your stir-fry vegetables and cook them together until they are tender. 4. Add broccoli to your omelets: Broccoli adds a delicious crunch and flavor to omelets. Simply chop up some broccoli and add it to your omelet mix. 5. Roast broccoli: Roasting broccoli is another easy and tasty way to incorporate it into your diet. Simply chop up the broccoli into florets, toss them with some olive oil, salt, and pepper, and roast them in the oven until they are tender and slightly crispy. Incorporating broccoli into your diet is a great way to boost your health and enjoy delicious meals at the same time.

The Incredible Health Benefits of Eating Garlic Regularly: What Science Says.

Garlic has been used for centuries as a natural remedy to treat a variety of ailments. It is known for its strong and pungent aroma, which adds a distinct flavor to various cuisines around the world. But did you know that garlic also has numerous health benefits? Recent scientific studies have confirmed that garlic is loaded with numerous bioactive compounds that can help improve your health in many ways. From reducing blood pressure and cholesterol levels to strengthening the immune system and fighting infections, garlic has been shown to be an incredibly powerful natural medicine. In this article, we'll explore the incredible health benefits of eating garlic regularly, and explore some simple ways to incorporate this superfood into your diet.

1. The Nutritional Value of Garlic

Garlic is a small but mighty superfood that has been used for thousands of years for both culinary and medicinal purposes. It is an excellent source of vitamins and minerals, including vitamin B6, vitamin C, and manganese, and it also contains small amounts of other important nutrients such as calcium, potassium, and selenium. One of the most important components of garlic is allicin, a sulfur-containing compound that is responsible for the pungent smell and many of the health benefits associated with garlic. Allicin has been shown to have antibacterial, antiviral, and antifungal properties, making it an effective natural remedy for a wide range of health problems. Garlic is also high in antioxidants, which protect the body from damaging free radicals and may help reduce the risk of chronic diseases such as cancer and heart disease. Additionally, garlic has been shown to have anti-inflammatory properties, which can help reduce inflammation and swelling in the body. Overall, garlic is an incredibly nutritious and health-promoting food that is easy to incorporate into your diet.

2. Garlic's Role in Boosting Immunity

Garlic is a well-known ingredient in many dishes around the world. This flavorful and pungent bulb has been used for centuries for its medicinal properties. One of the most significant health benefits of garlic is its ability to boost the immune system. Garlic contains compounds that enhance the immune system's function, making it more effective at fighting off bacteria, viruses, and other harmful microorganisms. Studies have shown that consuming garlic regularly can boost the production of white blood cells, which are essential for fighting infections and diseases. Garlic also contains compounds that have antiviral properties, which can help fight off viruses like the common cold and flu. Garlic's immune-boosting properties can also help prevent chronic diseases. Studies have found that consuming garlic regularly can reduce the risk of developing certain types of cancers, including stomach and colon cancer. Garlic can also help lower cholesterol levels and reduce the risk of heart disease. To reap the benefits of garlic's immune-boosting properties, it is recommended to consume it raw or lightly cooked. Cooking garlic can destroy some of its beneficial compounds, so it is best to use it as a seasoning or add it to dishes at the end of the cooking process. Overall, garlic is an excellent addition to any diet for its immune-boosting properties and numerous other health benefits. Incorporating garlic into your meals can help keep your immune system healthy and strong, benefiting your overall health and well-being.

3. Garlic and Heart Health

Garlic has long been known for its numerous health benefits, and one of the most significant benefits is related to heart health. Studies have shown that consuming garlic regularly can help reduce the risk of heart disease. Garlic helps to lower high blood pressure, which is a significant risk factor for heart disease. High blood pressure can cause damage to the arteries and increase the risk of heart disease. Garlic contains compounds that help prevent the formation of blood clots, which can also lead to heart disease. Additionally, garlic has been shown to reduce cholesterol levels, which is another major risk factor for heart disease. Some studies have even suggested that garlic can help improve overall heart function. In conclusion, consuming garlic regularly can provide significant benefits to heart health. If you are looking for a natural way to improve your heart health, consider adding garlic to your diet. However, it is essential to consult your doctor before making any significant changes to your diet.

4. Garlic and Cancer Prevention

There is a growing body of evidence that suggests that eating garlic regularly can help prevent cancer. Garlic contains compounds like allicin, diallyl sulfide, and allyl cysteine, which have been shown to have anti-cancer properties. These compounds work by boosting the immune system, inhibiting cancer cell growth, and reducing inflammation in the body. Studies have shown that people who eat garlic regularly have a reduced risk of several types of cancer, including stomach, colon, and pancreatic cancer. In fact, a study conducted by the National Cancer Institute found that people who ate garlic at least twice a week had a 44% lower risk of developing colon cancer than those who did not eat garlic. Additionally, a study conducted in China found that women who ate raw garlic at least once a week had a 35% lower risk of developing ovarian cancer. While more research is needed to fully understand how garlic affects cancer prevention, the evidence we have so far is promising. Eating garlic regularly is a simple and delicious way to potentially reduce your risk of developing cancer.

Why Brussel Sprouts Should Be Your New Favorite Vegetable: The Surprising Health Benefits.

When it comes to eating vegetables, many of us tend to stick to the same few we know and like. However, there is one vegetable that is often overlooked but deserves much more attention - brussel sprouts. These tiny, green vegetables may not be on everyone's favorite list, but they are packed with a surprising number of health benefits that make them one of the best vegetables you can add to your diet. From being loaded with vitamins and minerals to helping prevent chronic diseases, brussel sprouts have a lot to offer. In this article, we'll take a closer look at why brussel sprouts should be your new favorite vegetable and how you can start incorporating them into your meals today.

1. Introduction to Brussel Sprouts

Brussel sprouts are a vegetable that many people love to hate. They have a distinct flavor and odor that can be off-putting to some. However, if you haven't given Brussel sprouts a chance, you might be missing out on some incredible health benefits. Brussel sprouts are a member of the cruciferous vegetable family, which also includes broccoli, cauliflower, and kale. They are a low-calorie vegetable that is packed with nutrients, including vitamin C, vitamin K, and fiber. Brussel sprouts are also a great source of phytonutrients, which are natural compounds found in plants that have been shown to have anti-inflammatory and cancer-fighting properties. In this blog post, we will explore the many health benefits of Brussel sprouts and why you should consider making them a regular part of your diet.

2. Nutritional Benefits of Brussel Sprouts

Brussel sprouts are packed with important nutrients that your body needs to stay healthy. One of the most significant benefits of Brussel sprouts is their high fiber content. Eating just one cup of Brussel sprouts provides you with over 4 grams of fiber, which helps to keep your digestive system running smoothly. Additionally, Brussel sprouts are a great source of vitamin C, an important antioxidant that helps to protect your cells from damage. This antioxidant is also essential for healthy skin and a strong immune system. Brussel sprouts are also an excellent source of vitamin K, which is important for healthy bones and blood clotting. They contain a significant amount of folate, a B-vitamin that is important for healthy cell growth and development. Furthermore, Brussel sprouts are also a good source of iron, which is essential for healthy blood cells. With all of these nutritional benefits, it's easy to see why Brussel sprouts should be your new favorite vegetable.

3. Health Benefits of Brussel Sprouts

Brussel sprouts are a member of the cabbage family and are often overlooked as a vegetable choice. However, they are loaded with nutrients and have a surprising amount of health benefits. One of the most significant benefits of Brussel sprouts is their high vitamin C content, which is essential for a strong immune system. They are also an excellent source of vitamin K, which helps to maintain healthy bones. Additionally, Brussel sprouts are rich in fiber, which can help to lower cholesterol and promote healthy digestion. They also contain antioxidants, such as vitamin A, which can protect against cellular damage and reduce the risk of cancer. Brussel sprouts are also high in folate, a B vitamin that is essential for brain function, and can help to reduce the risk of depression. Finally, Brussel sprouts are low in calories and carbohydrates, which makes them a great choice for anyone looking to maintain a healthy weight. With so many health benefits, Brussel sprouts are definitely worth adding to your diet!

4. How to Cook Brussel Sprouts

Brussel sprouts are a very versatile vegetable, and there are many ways to cook them to bring out their unique flavor. First, you should choose fresh and firm brussel sprouts from your local grocery store or farmers market. Then, you can try roasting them in the oven with a little olive oil, salt, and pepper until they are crispy and caramelized. Another popular way to cook brussel sprouts is to sauté them with garlic and onions in a skillet until they are tender and slightly browned. You can also steam brussel sprouts and top them with a little butter or a light dressing. One of my favorite ways to eat brussel sprouts is to shave them into thin slices and use them as a base for a salad. They add a great crunch and nutty flavor to any dish. No matter how you choose to cook brussel sprouts, these little vegetables are packed with nutrients like vitamin K, vitamin C, and fiber, making them an excellent addition to any diet.

The Incredible Health Benefits of Eating Swiss Chard: What You Need to Know!

Eating healthy is essential for living a healthy life. While we all know we need to eat more vegetables, it can be difficult to know which ones to choose. Swiss chard is a superfood that has numerous health benefits that are often overlooked. This leafy green vegetable is packed with nutrients that can help lower your risk of heart disease, diabetes, and certain types of cancer. It is also a great source of vitamins and minerals that can help improve your overall health and wellbeing. In this article, we will explore the incredible health benefits of eating Swiss chard and how you can incorporate it into your diet to maintain a healthy lifestyle.

1. What is Swiss chard?
Swiss chard is a leafy green vegetable that is part of the beet family. It is also known as silverbeet, spinach beet, crab beet, bright lights, and seakale beet. Swiss chard is an excellent source of vitamins A, C, and K, as well as magnesium, potassium, iron, and fiber. The leaves of Swiss chard are green, and the stems are usually red, white, or yellow. Swiss chard is a versatile vegetable that can be eaten raw or cooked. It has a slightly bitter taste that is similar to spinach but with a more robust flavor. Swiss chard is often used in Mediterranean and Eastern European cuisine and is a popular ingredient in soups, stews, and salads. This leafy green vegetable is not only delicious, but it also has numerous health benefits that make it an excellent addition to a healthy diet. Whether you enjoy it raw in a salad or cooked in a favorite recipe, Swiss chard is a must-try vegetable that is sure to leave you feeling nourished and satisfied.

2. Nutritional benefits of Swiss chard
Swiss chard is a leafy green vegetable that is packed with essential nutrients. One cup of cooked Swiss chard contains only 35 calories and provides an impressive amount of vitamins and minerals. Swiss chard is an excellent source of vitamin K, vitamin A, and vitamin C. It also contains high amounts of magnesium, potassium, and iron. These essential nutrients help to support a healthy body and can also help to prevent chronic diseases such as heart disease and cancer. Swiss chard is also a good source of dietary fiber, which can help to promote healthy digestion and prevent constipation. Additionally, Swiss chard is rich in antioxidants that can help to protect the body against oxidative stress and inflammation. These antioxidants can also help to promote healthy skin and reduce the risk of chronic diseases. Another significant benefit of consuming Swiss chard is its low glycemic index. This means that it is an excellent food choice for individuals with diabetes or those looking to manage their blood sugar levels. Swiss chard has a low glycemic index, which means that it causes a slow and steady rise in blood sugar levels, helping to keep you feeling full and satisfied for longer periods. Overall, Swiss chard is an incredibly nutritious and healthy food choice. It is packed with essential nutrients, dietary fiber, and antioxidants, making it an excellent addition to any diet.

3. Health benefits of Swiss chard
Swiss chard is a leafy green vegetable that is packed with nutrients and health benefits. Here are just a few of the health benefits that come along with eating Swiss chard: 1. Lowers Blood Pressure: Swiss chard is high in potassium, a mineral that helps to lower blood pressure. It has been shown to be effective in reducing the risk of heart disease and stroke. 2. Rich in Antioxidants: Swiss chard is also rich in antioxidants, which help to protect the body from the damaging effects of free radicals. This can help to reduce the risk of cancer and other diseases. 3. Anti-Inflammatory: Swiss chard contains a variety of anti-

inflammatory compounds that can help to reduce inflammation in the body. This can help to reduce the risk of chronic diseases such as arthritis, diabetes, and heart disease. 4. Good for Digestion: Swiss chard is high in fiber, which is essential for good digestion. It can help to keep the digestive system running smoothly and can even help to prevent constipation. 5. Promotes Healthy Bones: Swiss chard is a good source of calcium, which is important for strong and healthy bones. It also contains vitamin K, which helps to promote bone health. Overall, Swiss chard is a delicious and nutritious vegetable that offers a wide range of health benefits. So the next time you're at the grocery store, be sure to pick up some Swiss chard and start reaping the benefits of this amazing food!

4. How to incorporate Swiss chard into your diet
Swiss chard is a leafy green vegetable that is packed with essential vitamins and nutrients. It's a great addition to any diet, and there are a variety of ways to incorporate it into your meals. One of the easiest ways to add Swiss chard to your diet is to simply chop it up and add it to your salads. Not only does it add a great flavor and texture, but it also provides a boost of nutrients to your meal. Swiss chard can also be sautéed with garlic and olive oil, providing a delicious and healthy side dish. Another way to incorporate Swiss chard is to use it as a substitute for spinach in recipes. It can be added to soups, stews, and casseroles, as well as being used as a topping for pizzas and flatbreads. If you're feeling adventurous, you can also make Swiss chard chips by baking the leaves in the oven. There are so many ways to add Swiss chard to your diet, and with its incredible health benefits, it's definitely worth incorporating into your meals.

The Amazing Benefits of Eating Beets: Why You Should Add Beets to Your Diet.

Beets are one of the most underrated and underutilized vegetables in the world today. They are often overlooked in favor of more popular vegetables like broccoli or carrots. However, beets contain an abundance of nutrients that can offer numerous benefits to your body. They are a good source of fiber, vitamin C, and essential minerals like potassium and manganese. Beets are also packed with antioxidants, which can help protect your cells from damage caused by free radicals. In this article, we'll explore the many amazing benefits of eating beets and provide you with some simple and delicious ways to add them to your diet. Whether you're looking to improve your heart health, boost your energy levels, or simply enjoy a delicious and nutritious vegetable, beets are definitely worth adding to your daily diet.

1. What are beets?

Beets are a root vegetable that are often overlooked, but they are incredibly nutritious and delicious. They are known for their deep red color and sweet taste, and they are a great source of essential vitamins and minerals. Beets are also a good source of dietary fiber, which can help regulate digestion and keep you feeling full for longer periods of time. This root vegetable is rich in vitamin C, which helps boost the immune system and reduce inflammation in the body. They also contain essential minerals like iron, magnesium, and potassium, all of which are important for maintaining healthy bodily functions. Beets are a versatile vegetable that can be cooked in a variety of ways, including roasting, boiling, or juicing. They can be eaten raw as well, the tops of the beetroot are edible and can be enjoyed in a salad or as a sautéed side dish. In summary, beets are a nutrient-rich root vegetable that can be a delicious and healthy addition to anyone's diet.

2. The nutritional value of beets

Beets are a root vegetable that are packed with nutrients and health benefits. They are known to be excellent sources of fiber, folate, vitamin C, potassium, and manganese. In addition, beets contain a high concentration of nitrates, which can help to improve blood pressure and boost exercise performance. One of the most impressive aspects of beets is their high concentration of antioxidants. These molecules help to reduce the damage caused by free radicals in the body, which can lead to chronic diseases like cancer and heart disease. Beets contain a variety of antioxidants, including betalains, which are associated with a reduced risk of chronic diseases. Beets are also known to have anti-inflammatory properties. Chronic inflammation is linked to a range of health problems, including arthritis, heart disease, and cancer. By eating beets, you can help to reduce inflammation in the body and prevent these conditions from developing. Finally, beets have been shown to improve cognitive function. This is due to their high concentration of nitrates, which help to increase blood flow to the brain. By improving blood flow, beets can help to boost memory, focus, and overall cognitive function. Overall, beets are a highly nutritious and beneficial food that should be included in any healthy diet.

3. Health benefits of eating beets

Beets are a root vegetable that has been gaining popularity in recent years for their numerous health benefits. They are a rich source of antioxidants, fiber, and essential vitamins and minerals. Eating beets has been linked to a range of health benefits, including lower blood pressure, improved digestion, and improved athletic performance. Beets are also a great source of dietary nitrates, which can improve blood flow and lower the risk of heart disease. In addition, the high levels of folate found in beets can support healthy brain function and reduce the risk of birth defects in pregnant women. Beets are also low in calories and high in fiber, making them an excellent choice for weight loss and weight management. Incorporating beets into your diet is easy and can be done in a variety of ways. You can roast them, steam them, or add them to salads and smoothies. So whether you're looking to improve your overall health or simply looking for a tasty new vegetable to add to your meals, beets are an excellent choice.

4. Ways to add beets to your diet.
If you're convinced that beets are a must-have in your diet, but you're not sure how to incorporate them, then you're in the right place. There are many delicious ways to add beets to your diet. One way is to roast them. Roasting beets brings out their natural sweetness and makes them tender and flavorful. You can season them with salt, pepper, and herbs for added flavor. Another way to add beets to your diet is to make a beet salad. Simply toss roasted beets with greens and other vegetables of your choice for a colorful and healthy salad. You can also add beets to smoothies, juices, and even desserts. Beets are amazingly versatile and can be used in a variety of dishes. You can also juice beets for a quick and easy way to get all the benefits of this superfood. Finally, you can pickle beets for a tasty and healthy snack. With so many options, it's easy to add beets to your diet and enjoy all the amazing benefits they have to offer.

The Many Benefits of Eating Asparagus: Why You Should Add It to Your Diet.

Asparagus is a vegetable that is often overlooked in the produce aisle, but it's time to give it the attention it deserves. Not only is asparagus delicious, it's also incredibly good for you. With so many vitamins, minerals, and nutrients packed into each spear, there are plenty of reasons to add this vegetable to your diet. From aiding in digestion to boosting your immune system, this article will delve into the many benefits of eating asparagus and why you should consider incorporating it into your meals. Whether you love it roasted, grilled, or sautéed, this versatile vegetable is a great addition to any dish. So, read on to discover how asparagus can improve your health and well-being.

1. Nutritional value of asparagus

Asparagus is a tasty and nutritious vegetable that is packed with essential vitamins and minerals. It is low in calories and high in fiber, making it an excellent addition to any diet. One cup of asparagus contains only 27 calories, making it a perfect snack for anyone looking to lose weight. It is also an excellent source of vitamin K, which is essential for healthy bones and blood clotting. Asparagus is also rich in vitamin A, which is essential for healthy skin and vision. Additionally, it is an excellent source of vitamin C, which helps to boost the immune system and fight off infections. One cup of asparagus also contains a healthy dose of folate, which is vital for pregnant women. It helps to prevent birth defects and promotes healthy brain development in babies. Asparagus is also rich in potassium, which is essential for healthy blood pressure and heart function. It is also a good source of iron, which helps to prevent anemia and promote healthy red blood cells. Asparagus is also a good source of antioxidants, which help to protect the body from damage caused by free radicals. The antioxidants in asparagus can help to prevent chronic diseases such as cancer, heart disease, and Alzheimer's disease. Overall, asparagus is an incredibly healthy vegetable that should be included in any healthy diet.

2. Health benefits of eating asparagus

Asparagus is a superfood that is low in calories and high in nutrients. It is a great source of fiber, folate, vitamins A, C, E, and K, as well as chromium, a trace mineral that enhances insulin's ability to transport glucose from the bloodstream into cells. Moreover, asparagus is packed with antioxidants that help to prevent disease and reduce the risk of chronic health conditions such as cancer, heart disease, and diabetes. Additionally, asparagus contains compounds called saponins that have been shown to reduce inflammation throughout the body, helping to fight off infections and diseases such as arthritis. Asparagus is also known to be a natural diuretic that helps to flush toxins and excess fluids from the body, promoting healthy kidney function. And if all of that wasn't enough, asparagus is also a great source of prebiotics, which provide food for the good bacteria in your gut, helping to improve digestive health and immune function. Overall, incorporating asparagus into your diet can provide a wide range of health benefits that can help you to feel better and live a longer, happier life.

3. Ways to incorporate asparagus into your diet

Asparagus is a great addition to any diet as it is low in calories, high in fiber, and loaded with vitamins and minerals. If you're looking to incorporate more asparagus into your diet, there are many delicious ways to do so. One of the simplest ways to enjoy asparagus is to roast it in the oven with a little olive oil and a sprinkle of salt and pepper. This brings out its natural sweetness and makes for a delicious side dish. Another way to enjoy asparagus is to steam it and toss it with a little lemon juice and grated Parmesan cheese. This makes for a tasty and healthy snack or appetizer. For a more substantial meal, try adding asparagus to stir-fries, risottos, or pasta dishes. Asparagus is also a great addition to salads and wraps, adding crunch and flavor. Finally, you can even try juicing asparagus for a nutrient-packed drink. With so many ways to incorporate asparagus into your diet, there's no excuse not to give it a try!

4. Conclusion.

In conclusion, asparagus is an incredibly healthy and delicious vegetable that provides a wide range of benefits for your overall health and wellbeing. Whether you are looking to improve your digestion, fight inflammation, boost your immune system or simply add some variety to your diet, asparagus is an excellent choice. It is packed full of vitamins, minerals, and antioxidants that are essential for maintaining good health, and it is also incredibly versatile, making it a great addition to a wide range of dishes. So why not try adding some asparagus to your diet today and start reaping the many benefits that this wonderful vegetable has to offer?

The Incredible Health Benefits of Eating Red Cabbage You Need to Know!

Eating a balanced diet is important for a healthy lifestyle. While many of us are aware of the benefits of eating fruits and vegetables, there are some that are often overlooked. One such vegetable is red cabbage. Not only is it a colorful addition to your plate, but it also has numerous health benefits that you may not know about. Red cabbage is low in calories, high in nutrients, and packed full of antioxidants, vitamins, and minerals. In this article, we will delve into the incredible health benefits of red cabbage that you need to know. From boosting your immune system and reducing inflammation to aiding digestion and promoting heart health, read on to find out why this vegetable should be a staple in your diet.

1. Nutritional Value of Red Cabbage
Red cabbage is not only visually appealing but is also jam-packed with nutrients. It is a type of cruciferous vegetable, just like broccoli and kale, and is known for its health benefits. Red cabbage is low in calories, with only 22 calories per 100 grams. However, it is rich in vitamins and minerals, including vitamin C, vitamin K, vitamin A, and potassium. It is also an excellent source of fiber, which is important for digestion and maintaining healthy bowel movements. Additionally, red cabbage contains antioxidants, such as anthocyanins, which can help to reduce inflammation in the body and protect against chronic diseases such as heart disease and cancer. Another great thing about red cabbage is that it is versatile and can be cooked in a variety of ways. You can add it to soups, stir-fries, and salads or use it as a base for your coleslaw. Overall, incorporating red cabbage into your diet is a great way to boost your nutrient intake and support your overall health.

2. Antioxidant and Anti-Inflammatory Properties of Red Cabbage
Red cabbage is an amazing vegetable that is packed with nutrients and health benefits. One of the most notable health benefits of red cabbage is its high content of antioxidants and anti-inflammatory properties. Red cabbage contains a group of antioxidants called anthocyanins, which give it its distinctive purple color. These antioxidants help to protect the body against free radicals, which are unstable molecules that can cause inflammation and damage to cells. In addition, red cabbage also contains compounds that have anti-inflammatory properties. These compounds can help to reduce inflammation in the body and may be beneficial for people with conditions such as arthritis, asthma, and other inflammatory conditions. Eating red cabbage regularly may also help to reduce the risk of chronic diseases such as heart disease, cancer, and diabetes. Overall, red cabbage is a powerful vegetable that can provide many health benefits when incorporated into a balanced and healthy diet.

3. Red Cabbage and Digestive Health
Red cabbage is loaded with nutrients and antioxidants that are essential for our overall health. One of the most significant health benefits of red cabbage is its impact on digestive health. Red cabbage is an excellent source of fiber, which is essential for maintaining a healthy digestive system. A diet high in fiber can help regulate bowel movements, prevent constipation, and reduce the risk of colon cancer. Moreover, red cabbage contains compounds called glucosinolates that can improve digestion by promoting the production of digestive enzymes. These enzymes play a crucial role in breaking down food and ensuring that it is absorbed properly by the body. One of the most important glucosinolates found in red cabbage is sulforaphane. This compound has been shown to have anti-inflammatory properties that can help alleviate digestive issues such as bloating and gas. Sulforaphane can also help protect the stomach lining

from damage caused by the bacteria Helicobacter pylori. In addition to its health benefits, red cabbage is delicious and incredibly versatile. It can be eaten raw in salads, pickled, sautéed, or roasted in the oven. Adding red cabbage to your diet is an easy way to improve your digestive health while enjoying a tasty and nutritious vegetable.

4. Red Cabbage and Heart Health

Red cabbage is a nutrient-dense, low-calorie vegetable that is packed with a variety of health benefits. One of the most significant benefits of consuming red cabbage is its positive impact on heart health. This is because red cabbage is high in antioxidants, which help to protect the body against free radical damage. Free radicals are unstable molecules that can damage the cells in the body and contribute to the development of chronic diseases. Red cabbage is also an excellent source of vitamin C, which is an essential nutrient for heart health. Vitamin C helps to protect the lining of the arteries from damage and can help to lower blood pressure. High blood pressure is a significant risk factor for heart disease, so keeping blood pressure within a healthy range is critical for maintaining good heart health. In addition to being high in antioxidants and vitamin C, red cabbage is also an excellent source of fiber, which is essential for heart health. Fiber can help to lower cholesterol levels and reduce the risk of heart disease. Red cabbage is also low in calories and contains no fat, making it an ideal food for maintaining a healthy weight, another essential factor in maintaining good heart health. Overall, incorporating red cabbage into your diet is an excellent way to support heart health and promote overall wellness. Whether you enjoy it raw in salads or cooked in your favorite recipes, there are many delicious ways to incorporate this nutrient-packed vegetable into your daily diet.

Fire Up Your Health: Discovering the Benefits of Eating Jalapeno Pepper.

Spice up your life with the Jalapeno Pepper! Often used as a topping or garnish, the Jalapeno Pepper is a versatile vegetable with a surprising number of health benefits. From reducing inflammation and aiding in digestion to increasing your metabolism and boosting your immune system, Jalapeno Pepper is a nutrient powerhouse that can improve your overall health. If you're looking for a way to add some heat to your meals and improve your health at the same time, read on to discover the benefits of eating Jalapeno Pepper. We'll also provide some tips on how to incorporate this flavorful vegetable into your diet.

1. Introduction to Jalapeno Pepper
Jalapeno pepper is a type of chili pepper that is widely used in Mexican cuisine. It is known for its pungent and spicy flavor, which adds heat to any dish. Jalapeno pepper is not only a great addition to your meal for taste purposes but also has numerous health benefits. It is high in vitamins A and C, which are essential for maintaining good health. It also contains capsaicin, a compound that is known to have anti-inflammatory properties, making it an excellent addition to your diet. Furthermore, jalapeno pepper is known to increase your metabolism, which can help you burn calories more efficiently. It is also beneficial for your digestive system, as it can help prevent stomach ulcers and other gastrointestinal issues. If you're looking for a healthy and spicy addition to your meals, jalapeno pepper is an excellent choice. In this blog post, we will explore the many benefits of eating jalapeno pepper and how you can incorporate it into your diet.

2. Nutritional Benefits of Jalapeno Pepper
Jalapeno peppers are more than just a spicy addition to your favorite dishes. They are also packed with nutritional benefits that can help you maintain a healthy lifestyle. One of the most significant benefits of jalapeno peppers is their high concentration of vitamins and minerals. They are an excellent source of vitamin C, which can help boost your immune system and fight off illnesses. Jalapeno peppers are also rich in vitamin A, which helps maintain healthy vision and skin. Additionally, they contain antioxidants, which can help reduce your risk of chronic diseases like cancer and heart disease. Jalapeno peppers are also low in calories, making them an ideal option for those trying to lose weight. They contain capsaicin, a compound that has been found to help speed up metabolism and burn fat. In fact, studies have shown that consuming spicy foods like jalapeno peppers can help you feel fuller for longer periods, which can help you eat fewer calories throughout the day. In addition to their nutritional benefits, jalapeno peppers are also a great way to add flavor to your meals. They can be eaten raw or cooked and are a popular addition to dishes like salsas, stews, and salads. If you're not a fan of spicy foods, you can still enjoy the nutritional benefits of jalapeno peppers by adding just a small amount to your meals. Overall, jalapeno peppers are a tasty and nutritious addition to any diet.

3. Health Benefits of Jalapeno Pepper
Jalapeno peppers are a popular ingredient in many different dishes, but did you know that they also have numerous health benefits? Jalapenos contain capsaicin, which is a natural anti-inflammatory agent that can help to reduce pain and inflammation in the body. They are also rich in vitamin C, which is an essential nutrient that supports a healthy immune system. Additionally, jalapenos have been shown to boost metabolism and promote weight loss. This is because they contain a compound called capsaicin, which has been shown to increase the body's metabolic rate, leading to increased calorie burning. Moreover, they

also contain antioxidants that can help to protect the body against damage from free radicals. Jalapenos have also been shown to have antibacterial and antifungal properties, which can help to prevent infections and promote overall digestive health. Finally, they can help to reduce inflammation in the body, which can be beneficial for those with inflammatory conditions such as arthritis or asthma. Therefore, adding jalapeno pepper to your diet can provide a variety of health benefits that can improve your overall well-being.

4. How to Incorporate Jalapeno Pepper into Your Diet

If you're looking to add some spice to your life and benefit your health in the process, jalapeno peppers are a great place to start. They are low in calories, high in vitamin C, and contain capsaicin, a compound that has been shown to have anti-inflammatory and pain-relieving effects. But how do you incorporate jalapeno pepper into your diet? One easy way to start is to add chopped jalapeno peppers to your favorite dish. For example, you can sprinkle them on top of your salad or add them to your scrambled eggs in the morning. You can also make a jalapeno salsa or guacamole to eat with your favorite tortilla chips. Another option is to stuff jalapenos with cheese and bake them in the oven for a delicious and healthy appetizer. If you're feeling brave, you can even try eating jalapeno peppers raw, but be warned, they are quite spicy! No matter how you decide to incorporate jalapeno peppers into your diet, they are sure to add some flavor and health benefits to your meals.

Mushroom Power: Exploring the Health Benefits of Adding Mushrooms to Your Diet.

Mushrooms are a versatile ingredient that can be added to almost any dish. Not only do they add depth and flavor to food, but they also offer a wide range of health benefits that are often overlooked in our daily lives. From boosting the immune system to aiding in digestion, mushrooms have been used for centuries in traditional medicine to treat various ailments. Recent studies have shown that the nutritional value of mushrooms is higher than previously thought, making them a powerhouse ingredient in any dish. In this article, we'll explore the many health benefits of mushrooms and show you how to incorporate them into your diet in creative and delicious ways. Whether you're a vegetarian, vegan, or just looking to improve your overall health and wellbeing, read on to discover the power of mushrooms.

1. Introduction to the benefits of mushrooms
Mushrooms are a versatile and delicious ingredient that has been used in cooking for centuries. However, what many people don't know is that mushrooms are also packed with health benefits. These little fungi are a rich source of many essential nutrients, including vitamins B and D, selenium, potassium, and copper. They also contain powerful antioxidants that can help protect against cell damage and inflammation. Additionally, mushrooms have been shown to have anti-inflammatory, anti-tumor, and immune-boosting properties. They may also help regulate blood sugar levels, reduce cholesterol, and even improve mental health. With so many health benefits, it's no wonder that mushrooms are becoming increasingly popular as a food and supplement. Whether you are looking to improve your overall health or simply want to add variety to your diet, mushrooms are an excellent choice.

2. Nutritional value of mushrooms
Mushrooms are a low-calorie, high-fiber food that is also rich in vitamins and minerals. They are a great addition to any diet, whether you're a vegetarian, vegan, or a meat-eater. Mushrooms are low in calories and high in nutrients, which makes them an excellent food for weight loss. They also contain essential amino acids, which are the building blocks of protein. Mushrooms are also an excellent source of riboflavin, niacin, and selenium. Riboflavin helps to maintain healthy red blood cells, while niacin helps to keep the skin and digestive system healthy. Selenium is an antioxidant that helps to protect the body against damage from free radicals. Mushrooms are also a good source of potassium, which helps to regulate blood pressure and maintain healthy muscles and nerves. Additionally, mushrooms contain beta-glucans, which have been shown to have immunomodulatory and anticancer effects. All of these nutrients and health benefits make mushrooms a great addition to any diet.

3. Health benefits of mushrooms
Mushrooms are a fantastic and versatile food item that can be used in a variety of dishes. Not only are they delicious, but they are also packed full of health benefits that make them a great addition to any diet. One of the main benefits of mushrooms is that they are high in antioxidants, which are essential for maintaining a healthy immune system. They are also a good source of fiber, which is important for digestion and maintaining a healthy weight. Additionally, mushrooms are full of vitamins and minerals, including vitamin D, potassium, and selenium. These vitamins and minerals are essential for maintaining healthy skin, hair, nails, and bones. In fact, mushrooms are one of the few natural sources of vitamin D, making them an excellent addition to a vegan or vegetarian diet. The beta-glucans found in mushrooms are also known to have immune-boosting properties, helping to fight infections and illnesses. Finally,

mushrooms are low in calories and fat, making them an excellent food choice for those looking to lose weight or maintain a healthy lifestyle. With so many health benefits, it's no surprise that mushrooms are becoming increasingly popular as a food item.

4. How to incorporate mushrooms into your diet.
Mushrooms are a delicious and nutritious addition to any diet. They are versatile and can be used in many different ways, from soups and stews to salads and sandwiches. If you're looking to incorporate mushrooms into your diet, here are a few tips to get you started. First, consider trying different varieties of mushrooms. There are over 10,000 different types of mushrooms, each with their own unique flavor and nutritional benefits. Some popular varieties include button mushrooms, shiitake mushrooms, portobello mushrooms, and oyster mushrooms. Second, try adding mushrooms to your favorite recipes. For example, you can sauté mushrooms and add them to omelets or frittatas, chop them up and add them to pasta dishes, or even grill them and use them as a burger topping. Third, consider using mushrooms as a meat substitute in some of your favorite recipes. Mushrooms are a great source of protein and can be used in place of meat in many dishes, such as stir-fries or tacos. Finally, consider incorporating mushrooms into your diet by drinking mushroom tea or taking mushroom supplements. These products contain concentrated amounts of mushroom extracts and can be a convenient way to reap the health benefits of mushrooms. Incorporating mushrooms into your diet is easy and can provide a wide array of health benefits. Whether you're a seasoned mushroom lover or just starting to explore their culinary potential, there are many ways to enjoy these delicious and nutritious fungi.

The Amazing Health Benefits of Adding Butternut Squash to Your Diet.

Butternut squash may not be the first thing that comes to mind when you think of healthy foods, but it should be! This delicious and versatile vegetable is packed with nutrients that can provide numerous health benefits. It is rich in fiber, vitamins, and minerals that can help improve digestion, boost the immune system, and promote healthy skin and hair. The sweet and slightly nutty taste of butternut squash is perfect for adding depth to your meals. Whether you roast it, mash it, or turn it into a soup, this vegetable is sure to be a hit with the whole family. In this article, we'll take a closer look at the amazing health benefits of butternut squash and give you some delicious recipe ideas to incorporate it into your diet.

1. The nutritional value of butternut squash
Butternut squash is a popular winter squash that is known for its sweet, nutty flavor and versatility in cooking. But what many people may not know is that butternut squash is also incredibly nutritious. It is low in calories, high in fiber, and packed with essential vitamins and minerals. One cup of cooked butternut squash contains only around 80 calories and provides over 200% of your daily recommended intake of vitamin A, which is essential for maintaining healthy skin, vision, and immune function. Butternut squash is also a good source of vitamin C, potassium, magnesium, and other important nutrients that support overall health and well-being. In addition to its impressive nutritional profile, butternut squash is also rich in antioxidants. These powerful compounds help to protect the body from oxidative stress and inflammation, which are linked to a range of chronic health conditions, including heart disease, cancer, and diabetes. Overall, incorporating butternut squash into your diet is a great way to support your health and enjoy delicious, nourishing meals. Whether roasted, mashed, or pureed, this versatile winter squash is a great addition to soups, stews, salads, and more.

2. Health benefits of butternut squash
Butternut squash is a delicious and nutritious vegetable that is packed with numerous health benefits. One of the primary benefits of butternut squash is that it is rich in antioxidants. Antioxidants help to neutralize harmful free radicals in the body that cause cell damage and contribute to the development of chronic diseases such as cancer, heart disease, and Alzheimer's disease. Additionally, butternut squash is a good source of fiber, which can help to improve digestive health by promoting regular bowel movements and reducing the risk of constipation. This vegetable is also known to be rich in vitamin A and potassium. Vitamin A is essential for maintaining good vision, a healthy immune system, and skin health. It also helps to regulate cell growth and division, which is important for maintaining healthy skin and reducing the risk of certain types of cancer. Potassium is an essential mineral that helps to regulate fluid balance in the body, which can help to reduce the risk of high blood pressure, stroke, and heart disease. Moreover, butternut squash is low in calories and high in nutrients, making it an excellent choice for weight management. It is also a good source of vitamin C, which can help to boost the immune system and reduce the risk of chronic diseases. Overall, by adding butternut squash to your diet, you can benefit from its numerous health benefits and enjoy a delicious and nutritious vegetable that is easy to prepare and versatile in many dishes.

3. How to prepare butternut squash
If you're looking to add more butternut squash to your diet, you may be wondering how to prepare it. Luckily, butternut squash is a versatile vegetable that can be cooked in many different ways. Here are a

few ideas to get you started: 1. Roast butternut squash in the oven with a little olive oil and your favorite herbs and spices. This is a simple and tasty way to prepare the squash, and it can be used as a side dish or added to salads. 2. Make butternut squash soup. Simply boil the squash until it is soft, then blend it with some vegetable stock, onions, and garlic. This is a great way to get a lot of squash into your diet, especially if you're not a big fan of the taste. 3. Use butternut squash as a pasta sauce. Simply roast the squash with some garlic and olive oil, then blend it with some cream or milk to make a creamy sauce. This is a great way to add some extra nutrition to your pasta dishes. 4. Add butternut squash to your breakfast. Roast some squash with a little cinnamon and nutmeg, then add it to your oatmeal or yogurt for a healthy and delicious breakfast. No matter how you prepare it, adding butternut squash to your diet is a great way to improve your health and enjoy some tasty meals at the same time.

4. Delicious and healthy butternut squash recipe ideas.
Butternut squash is a delicious and healthy vegetable that can be added to a variety of dishes. It is a rich source of vitamins A and C, potassium, and fiber. Moreover, it is low in calories and fat, making it an excellent choice for those who are trying to maintain a healthy diet. If you're looking for some delicious and healthy ways to incorporate butternut squash into your diet, here are a few recipe ideas for you to try. 1. Butternut Squash Soup: A creamy and comforting soup that is perfect for chilly evenings. It is a simple recipe that only requires a few ingredients, including butternut squash, onion, garlic, and chicken or vegetable broth. 2. Roasted Butternut Squash: This is a simple recipe that requires only a few ingredients, including butternut squash, olive oil, salt, and pepper. Roasting the squash brings out its natural sweetness and makes it tender and delicious. 3. Butternut Squash Risotto: This is a creamy and delicious risotto that is perfect for a cozy night in. It requires a little bit of effort, but the end result is well worth it. 4. Butternut Squash and Kale Salad: This salad is a healthy and flavorful way to incorporate butternut squash into your diet. It is a mix of roasted butternut squash, kale, quinoa, and cranberries, topped with a maple dijon dressing. These are just a few of the many delicious and healthy ways to incorporate butternut squash into your diet. With its versatility and health benefits, it's no wonder why this vegetable is becoming a popular choice for many people.

From Jack-O-Lanterns to Superfoods: The Surprising Health Benefits of Pumpkin.

Pumpkins have been a symbol of Halloween for centuries, but did you know that they're also packed with essential vitamins and nutrients that can benefit your health in numerous ways? More than just a seasonal decoration or ingredient in your favorite pumpkin spice latte, pumpkins have a variety of health benefits that make them a superfood you'll want to incorporate into your diet year-round. From improving heart health and boosting immunity to aiding in weight loss and promoting healthy skin, pumpkins have a multitude of health benefits that are often overlooked. In this article, we'll explore the surprising health benefits of pumpkins and show you how to incorporate this versatile and nutritious food into your diet in delicious and easy ways.

1. The Nutritional Benefits of Pumpkin
Pumpkin is a versatile vegetable that is packed with essential nutrients. It is low in calories and high in fiber, making it a great option for those looking to maintain a healthy diet. Pumpkin is also rich in vitamins A, C, and E, as well as minerals like potassium and magnesium. These nutrients work together to boost the immune system, improve vision, and promote healthy skin. Additionally, pumpkin is a good source of antioxidants, which can help prevent cell damage caused by free radicals. Studies have also shown that consuming pumpkin can help regulate blood sugar levels, making it a great option for those with diabetes. Furthermore, pumpkin seeds are a great source of protein, healthy fats, and magnesium. They can be eaten on their own as a snack or added to salads or soups for extra nutrition. Overall, pumpkin is a delicious and nutritious vegetable that can be incorporated into a variety of dishes and provide numerous health benefits.

2. How Pumpkin Can Boost Your Immune System
Pumpkins are not only great for carving jack-o-lanterns, but they're also a fantastic source of nutrients that can help boost your immune system. Pumpkin contains a high amount of beta-carotene, an antioxidant that the body converts into vitamin A. This vitamin is essential for maintaining healthy skin, vision, and immune function. Pumpkin also contains plenty of vitamin C, an antioxidant that can help fight off infections and support the immune system. Additionally, pumpkins are rich in zinc, which is crucial for maintaining a healthy immune system. Zinc helps to protect against viruses and bacteria and also supports the body's ability to heal wounds. Furthermore, pumpkin seeds are packed with nutrients, including magnesium, zinc, and healthy fats, all of which play a role in supporting immune function. So, if you want to boost your immune system, consider incorporating pumpkin into your diet. It's easy to add pumpkin puree to smoothies, oatmeal, or even baked goods like muffins or bread. You can also roast pumpkin seeds for a healthy and delicious snack.

3. How Pumpkin Can Help With Weight Loss
Pumpkin is a nutrient-dense food that is low in calories and high in fiber. Because of this, it can be a great addition to a weight loss diet. First, the fiber in pumpkin helps you to feel full, which can prevent overeating and snacking between meals. Additionally, the high water content in pumpkin can help keep you hydrated, which is important for maintaining a healthy weight. Pumpkin is also loaded with vitamins and minerals that can help you to feel more energized and less likely to turn to high-calorie junk food for a quick energy boost. Finally, pumpkin seeds are an excellent source of protein, which can help you to build and maintain lean muscle mass. All of these factors make pumpkin a great choice for anyone looking

to lose weight in a healthy and sustainable way. So next time you're looking for a nutritious and low-calorie snack, consider reaching for some pumpkin!

4. Delicious Ways to Incorporate Pumpkin Into Your Diet.
Pumpkin is a versatile and delicious ingredient that can be used in a variety of dishes. Not only is it tasty, but it is also packed with nutrients that are beneficial for your health. Here are some delicious ways to incorporate pumpkin into your diet: 1. Pumpkin soup: Pumpkin soup is a comforting and healthy meal that is perfect for fall. It is easy to make, and you can add your favorite spices and herbs to make it even more flavorful. 2. Pumpkin smoothie: If you are looking for a healthy breakfast or snack, a pumpkin smoothie is a great option. Blend pumpkin puree, almond milk, Greek yogurt, and your favorite fruits to create a tasty and nutritious drink. 3. Pumpkin pasta: Pumpkin puree can be used to create a creamy and flavorful pasta sauce. Add some roasted vegetables or grilled chicken to make it a complete meal. 4. Pumpkin bread: Pumpkin bread is a delicious and healthy alternative to regular bread. You can make it with whole wheat flour and add nuts and seeds for some extra texture. 5. Pumpkin pie: Pumpkin pie is a classic fall dessert that can be made healthier by using a whole wheat crust and reducing the amount of sugar in the filling. Incorporating pumpkin into your diet is an easy and tasty way to boost your health and enjoy the flavors of fall.

The Surprising Health Benefits of Eating Red Bell Peppers.

When we think of healthy eating, bell peppers, particularly red bell peppers, might not be the first thing that comes to mind. However, this vibrant vegetable is actually packed with nutrients that can improve our overall health and wellbeing. Red bell peppers are a rich source of vitamins A, C and K, as well as antioxidants and fiber. They can help reduce inflammation, support healthy skin and eyes, and even aid in weight loss. In this article, we will explore the surprising health benefits of eating red bell peppers, and provide you with some delicious recipes to help you incorporate them into your diet.

1. Nutritional value of red bell peppers
Red bell peppers are not only delicious but also incredibly nutritious. They are a great source of vitamins A, C, and K, as well as fiber, potassium, and folate. Just one red bell pepper contains more than 100% of the recommended daily value of vitamin C, which is essential for healthy skin, immune function, and wound healing. Additionally, red bell peppers are low in calories, making them an excellent choice for those trying to maintain a healthy weight. But that's not all—red bell peppers also contain powerful antioxidants that can help protect the body from damage caused by free radicals. These antioxidants are especially important for maintaining heart health and reducing the risk of chronic diseases, such as cancer and diabetes. So not only are red bell peppers a tasty addition to your diet, but they can also provide a range of health benefits that can help you feel your best.

2. Health benefits of eating red bell peppers
Red bell peppers are a great addition to any diet. Not only do they add a pop of color and flavor to dishes, but they are also packed with nutrients that can benefit your health. Here are just a few of the health benefits of eating red bell peppers: 1. High in Vitamin C - Red bell peppers contain a high amount of vitamin C, which can help boost your immune system and keep you healthy. 2. Helps with Digestion - The fiber in red bell peppers can help keep your digestive system running smoothly and prevent constipation. 3. Rich in Antioxidants - Red bell peppers are also rich in antioxidants, which can help protect your cells from damage caused by free radicals. 4. Low in Calories - Red bell peppers are low in calories, making them a great snack or addition to any meal for those looking to maintain or lose weight. 5. Can Improve Eye Health - Red bell peppers contain a high amount of vitamin A, which is essential for eye health and can help prevent vision loss. Overall, red bell peppers are a tasty and nutritious addition to any diet, offering a wide range of health benefits.

3. How to incorporate red bell peppers into your diet
Red bell peppers are a healthy and delicious addition to any diet. They are packed with vitamins, minerals, and antioxidants that can help boost your immune system and promote healthy skin and eyes. But how can you incorporate them into your diet? Here are a few simple ways to get more red bell peppers into your meals: 1. Add them to salads: Red bell peppers add a sweet and crunchy texture to salads. Simply chop them up and add them to your favorite greens. 2. Roast them: Roasting red bell peppers brings out their natural sweetness and makes them a great addition to any dish. Roast them in the oven or on the grill and use them in pasta dishes, sandwiches, or as a topping for pizza. 3. Use them as a dip: Red bell peppers are perfect for making dips like hummus or salsa. Simply blend them with other ingredients like chickpeas or tomatoes for a healthy and flavorful snack. 4. Stuff them: Red bell peppers can be stuffed with a variety of ingredients, like quinoa, beans, or ground turkey. This makes for a healthy and filling meal that is sure to satisfy. By incorporating red bell peppers into your diet, you're not only adding a burst of flavor to your meals, but you're also reaping the many health benefits they have to offer.

4. Delicious red bell pepper recipes.
Red bell peppers are a great addition to any meal, and they come with a variety of health benefits. Not only are they low in calories and high in nutrients, but they also contain powerful antioxidants that can help to fight inflammation and chronic diseases. If you're looking for some delicious ways to incorporate red bell peppers into your diet, here are a few recipe ideas to get you started: 1. Red Bell Pepper Soup: This creamy soup is perfect for a chilly day. Simply sauté some onions and garlic in olive oil, add chopped red bell peppers and vegetable broth, and let it simmer until the peppers are tender. Blend the mixture until it's smooth, and then add a dollop of cream or coconut milk for extra richness. 2. Stuffed Red Bell Peppers: Cut the tops off of some red bell peppers and remove the seeds and membranes. Fill them with a mixture of cooked rice, ground beef or turkey, chopped onions, and diced tomatoes. Bake them in the oven until the peppers are tender and the filling is hot and bubbly. 3. Red Bell Pepper Stir-Fry: Cut some red bell peppers into thin strips and stir-fry them with your favorite vegetables and protein. Season with soy sauce, garlic, and ginger, and serve over rice or noodles for a delicious and healthy meal. Whether you're looking for a hearty soup, a savory stuffed pepper, or a fresh and flavorful stir-fry, there are endless ways to enjoy the health benefits of red bell peppers.

Radicchio: The Superfood You Should Be Eating Today!

Eating healthy is important, but sometimes it can be difficult to know which foods are truly beneficial for our health. One superfood that you may not have heard of yet is radicchio. This leafy vegetable is not only packed with vitamins and minerals, but it also has a distinct and delicious flavor that can add variety to any meal. In this article, we will dive into the health benefits of radicchio and provide some creative and easy ways to incorporate it into your diet. So if you're looking to add something new and healthy to your meals, read on to discover why radicchio is the superfood you should be eating today!

1. What is radicchio?
Radicchio is a type of vegetable that belongs to the chicory family. It is often used in salads and has a slightly bitter taste. Radicchio is known for its deep red color, which makes it an attractive addition to any dish. It is also low in calories and high in antioxidants, making it a superfood that you should definitely be eating today. Radicchio is a great source of vitamins and minerals, including vitamin K, vitamin C, and folate. Additionally, it contains polyphenols, which are plant compounds that have been shown to have anti-inflammatory properties. This makes it a great vegetable for reducing inflammation in the body and promoting overall health. Radicchio is also a good source of dietary fiber, which can help keep you feeling full and satisfied after eating. It is a versatile vegetable that can be prepared in a variety of ways, including grilling, roasting, and sauteing. So, if you're looking for a nutritious and delicious vegetable to add to your diet, try incorporating some radicchio into your meals today!

2. Nutritional benefits of radicchio
Radicchio is a leafy vegetable that is gaining popularity for its numerous health benefits. This superfood is packed with nutrients that can help improve your overall health. Some of the nutritional benefits of radicchio include high levels of vitamin K, C, and B vitamins. Vitamin K is essential for bone health, while vitamin C helps support a healthy immune system. B vitamins are also critical for energy production and maintaining a healthy nervous system. Radicchio is also a great source of antioxidants, including polyphenols, anthocyanins, and flavonoids. These antioxidants can help protect the body against free radicals and reduce the risk of chronic diseases such as cancer, heart disease, and diabetes. Additionally, radicchio contains dietary fiber, which is critical for digestive health and can help lower cholesterol levels. Finally, radicchio is low in calories, making it an excellent option for those trying to lose weight or maintain a healthy weight. Overall, radicchio is a nutrient-packed vegetable that can help improve your overall health and well-being.

3. How to prepare and cook radicchio
Radicchio is a delicious vegetable that can add a lot of flavor and nutrition to your meals. However, if you've never prepared or cooked radicchio before, it can be a little intimidating. Here are some tips to help you get started. First, you'll want to select a fresh head of radicchio from the grocery store or farmer's market. Look for bright red leaves that are firm and crisp. Next, rinse the radicchio under cold water and pat it dry with a paper towel. To prepare the radicchio, you'll want to remove the bitter core. Simply cut the head in half lengthwise and use a sharp knife to carefully cut out the core. Once the core is removed, you can slice the radicchio into thin strips or chop it into bite-sized pieces. Radicchio can be eaten raw or cooked. If you're eating it raw, you can add it to salads, sandwiches, or wraps. It's also delicious when paired with ingredients like goat cheese, walnuts, or balsamic vinaigrette. If you're cooking radicchio, you can sauté it in a pan with a little olive oil and garlic. Cook it over medium heat for a few minutes until it's slightly wilted and caramelized. You can also roast radicchio in the oven with other vegetables for a side

dish. Overall, radicchio is a versatile and tasty superfood that can add a lot of nutrition and flavor to your meals. Don't be afraid to experiment with different preparation and cooking methods to find your favorite way to enjoy this delicious vegetable!

4. Creative recipes incorporating radicchio

Radicchio is a versatile and nutritious superfood that can be used in a variety of creative recipes. It has a slightly bitter taste, which makes it perfect for adding flavor and texture to salads or sandwiches. One delicious and simple way to incorporate radicchio into your diet is to make a salad with mixed greens, avocado, and orange slices. Toss in some toasted nuts, such as almonds or walnuts, and dress it with a citrus vinaigrette. Another creative recipe that incorporates radicchio is a grilled radicchio salad with goat cheese and figs. Simply grill the radicchio until it is slightly charred, then top it with crumbled goat cheese, sliced figs, and a drizzle of balsamic vinegar. This dish is perfect for a summer barbecue or a dinner party. Radicchio can also be used as a flavorful and nutritious topping for pizzas. Simply chop it into small pieces and sprinkle it on top of your favorite pizza toppings. It pairs well with ingredients such as prosciutto, mushrooms, and roasted garlic. Additionally, radicchio can be cooked as a side dish. Sauté it with garlic and olive oil until it is tender, and then serve it alongside a grilled steak or roasted chicken. With these creative recipes, you will be able to enjoy the delicious and nutritious benefits of radicchio in a variety of ways.

Incredible Health Benefits of Adding Endive to Your Diet.

If you're looking for a new vegetable to add to your diet, consider endive. This often-overlooked leafy green is actually packed with nutrients and offers a variety of health benefits. Not only is it low in calories, but it's also high in fiber, vitamins, and minerals. Endive contains vitamins C, K, and A, as well as folate, potassium, and manganese. It's also high in antioxidants, which can help to protect your cells from damage caused by free radicals. In this article, we'll take a closer look at some of the incredible health benefits of adding endive to your diet, along with some delicious and easy ways to incorporate it into your meals.

1. What is endive?
Endive is a leafy vegetable that is often used in salads or as a healthy snack. It has a slightly bitter taste and is commonly known as chicory in some parts of the world. Endive is a great source of vitamins and minerals, including Vitamin C, Vitamin K, and Folate. It is also low in calories and high in fiber, making it an excellent choice for those looking to maintain a healthy diet. Endive is a member of the lettuce family and can be found in many different varieties, including curly endive, Belgian endive, and escarole. It is a versatile ingredient that can be eaten raw, cooked, or grilled, and can be used in a variety of different dishes. With its unique flavor and incredible health benefits, endive is a great addition to any diet.

2. Nutritional benefits of endive
Endive is a leafy vegetable that is often overlooked in the produce section, but it is a powerhouse of nutrition. It is a great addition to any diet as it is low in calories and high in fiber. Endive is also a rich source of vitamins and minerals, including vitamin A, vitamin K, folate, and potassium. One of the most significant benefits of endive is its high fiber content. A single cup of raw endive contains around 3 grams of dietary fiber, which is almost 10% of the recommended daily intake. Fiber is essential for maintaining digestive health and can help prevent constipation and other digestive disorders. Endive is also rich in vitamin A, which is essential for healthy eyesight, the immune system, and skin health. It is also a great source of vitamin K, which is important for blood clotting and bone health. Additionally, endive contains folate, which is essential for cell growth and repair and helps to prevent birth defects. Endive is also an excellent source of potassium, which is essential for maintaining healthy blood pressure and preventing heart disease. It is also low in sodium, making it an ideal food for people on a low-sodium diet. Overall, endive is a flavorful and nutritious addition to any diet. Whether you are looking to improve your digestive health, boost your immune system, or prevent chronic diseases, adding endive to your diet is an easy and delicious way to do so.

3. Health benefits of endive
Endive is a nutrient-dense vegetable that is packed with vitamins, minerals, and antioxidants. Here are some of the incredible health benefits of adding endive to your diet: 1. Endive is rich in vitamins and minerals: Endive is a great source of vitamins A, K, and C, as well as folate, potassium, and calcium. These vitamins and minerals are essential for maintaining healthy bones, skin, and eyesight, as well as for supporting a healthy immune system. 2. Endive is high in fiber: Endive is a great source of dietary fiber, which is essential for maintaining a healthy digestive system. Fiber can help prevent constipation and other digestive problems, and can also help you feel full for longer periods of time, which can aid in weight loss. 3. Endive is low in calories: Endive is a great addition to a low-calorie diet, as it is very low in calories. This means that you can eat a large amount of endive without consuming too many calories, helping you maintain a healthy weight. 4. Endive is a good source of antioxidants: Endive is high in antioxidants, which are important for protecting your body against damage from harmful free radicals.

Antioxidants help prevent chronic diseases and can also help reduce inflammation in the body. Overall, adding endive to your diet is a great way to boost your nutrient intake and improve your overall health. Whether you enjoy it raw in a salad or cooked in a delicious recipe, endive is a versatile and nutritious vegetable that is worth adding to your diet.

4. Ways to incorporate endive into your diet.
Endive is an incredibly healthy vegetable that is packed with essential vitamins, minerals, and nutrients that our bodies need. However, many people are not sure how to incorporate it into their diets. Here are some simple ways to add endive to your diet: 1. In salads: Endive leaves are great for adding a fresh crunch to salads. You can chop them up and mix them with your favorite greens, veggies, and dressing. 2. As a snack: Endive leaves can be used as a healthy and crunchy snack. You can add hummus, salsa, or other dips to give them extra flavor. 3. In smoothies: Endive can be added to smoothies for a boost of nutrients. It pairs well with fruits like bananas, apples, and berries. 4. Grilled: Grilled endive is a delicious and healthy side dish. You can brush it with olive oil and sprinkle it with herbs for added flavor. 5. In soups: Endive can be added to soups for a fresh crunch and a boost of nutrients. It pairs well with other veggies like carrots, celery, and onions. Incorporating endive into your diet is a great way to improve your overall health and well-being. Try out these simple ways to add endive to your meals and enjoy the many health benefits it has to offer.

The Power of Cauliflower: Surprising Health Benefits You Need to Know.

Cauliflower is a versatile and delicious vegetable that can be used in many different ways in the kitchen. But did you know that it is also incredibly beneficial for your health? This cruciferous vegetable is packed with vitamins, minerals, and antioxidants that can help to improve your overall well-being. From reducing the risk of cancer and heart disease to promoting healthy digestion and boosting brain function, the health benefits of cauliflower are truly amazing. In this article, we will take a closer look at some of the surprising health benefits of cauliflower that you need to know about. Whether you are looking to improve your diet or simply want to learn more about the health benefits of this amazing vegetable, this article is for you.

1. What is cauliflower?

Cauliflower is a versatile and nutritious vegetable that belongs to the same family as broccoli, kale, and cabbage. It is known for its white, dense, and tightly packed florets that form a compact head, also known as a "curd." The cauliflower curd is surrounded by thick green leaves that protect it from direct sunlight. Cauliflower is usually available in white, but it can also be found in other colors such as green, purple, and orange. It is a great source of vitamins, minerals, and antioxidants, making it an excellent choice for people who are looking for a healthy and nutritious diet. The best part about cauliflower is that it is very low in calories and carbs, making it a great choice for those who are watching their weight or trying to eat low-carb diets. If you haven't tried cauliflower yet, I highly recommend giving it a try. You'll be amazed at how versatile and delicious it can be!

2. Nutritional benefits of cauliflower

Cauliflower is an incredible vegetable that's packed with important nutrients that our bodies need. One of the most significant nutritional benefits of cauliflower is that it is rich in vitamins and minerals. It is an excellent source of vitamin C, vitamin K, folate, and vitamin B6. Additionally, it contains many essential minerals like potassium, magnesium, and phosphorus, which are essential for maintaining a healthy body. Another significant benefit of cauliflower is that it is low in calories and high in fiber. A mere cup of raw cauliflower contains only about 25 calories, making it an excellent choice for those who are trying to lose weight. Additionally, the high fiber content in cauliflower helps promote healthy digestion and can help protect against certain types of cancer. Cauliflower is also a great source of antioxidants, which are essential for protecting our bodies against harmful free radicals. These free radicals can cause damage to our cells, leading to premature aging, cancer, and other diseases. Antioxidants help neutralize these free radicals and prevent this damage from occurring. Finally, cauliflower is a versatile vegetable that can be used in a variety of dishes. It can be roasted, steamed, mashed, or even used as a pizza crust or rice substitute. Whether you are looking to improve your health, lose weight, or simply enjoy a delicious and nutritious meal, cauliflower is an excellent choice that offers incredible health benefits.

3. Health benefits of cauliflower

Cauliflower is a cruciferous vegetable that is low in calories and high in nutrients. It is packed with vitamins, minerals, and antioxidants that provide numerous health benefits. Some of the health benefits of cauliflower include: 1. Boosts Immunity: Cauliflower contains high levels of vitamin C, which helps to boost the immune system and fight off infections. 2. Promotes Digestive Health: The fiber in cauliflower helps to improve digestion and reduce the risk of constipation and other digestive issues. 3. Reduces Inflammation: Cauliflower is rich in antioxidants such as quercetin and kaempferol, which help to reduce inflammation in the body and lower the risk of chronic diseases. 4. Supports Heart Health: The fiber and antioxidants in cauliflower help to promote heart health by reducing cholesterol levels and improving blood flow. 5. May Help Prevent Cancer: Cauliflower contains compounds such as sulforaphane and indole-3-carbinol, which have been shown to have anti-cancer properties and may help prevent certain types of cancer. Overall, cauliflower is a nutritious and delicious vegetable that offers a variety of health benefits. It can be enjoyed raw, roasted, grilled, or steamed, making it a versatile addition to any diet.

4. Creative ways to incorporate cauliflower into your diet.
Cauliflower is a versatile vegetable that can be used in many different ways. Incorporating cauliflower into your diet can be an excellent way to improve your health and add variety to your meals. Here are some creative ways to incorporate cauliflower into your diet: 1. Roasted cauliflower: Roasting cauliflower is a great way to bring out its natural sweetness. Simply cut the cauliflower into small florets, toss them in olive oil, and roast them in the oven until they are tender and golden brown. 2. Cauliflower rice: Cauliflower rice is a low-carb and grain-free alternative to traditional rice. To make cauliflower rice, simply pulse cauliflower florets in a food processor until they are the size of rice grains. Then, sauté the cauliflower rice in a pan with some olive oil and your favorite seasonings. 3. Cauliflower pizza crust: Cauliflower pizza crust is a delicious and healthy alternative to traditional pizza crust. To make cauliflower pizza crust, simply pulse cauliflower florets in a food processor until they are the size of rice grains. Then, add some almond flour, egg, and your favorite seasonings, and bake in the oven. 4. Cauliflower mash: Cauliflower mash is a great low-carb alternative to mashed potatoes. Simply boil cauliflower florets until they are tender, then mash them with some butter, cream, and your favorite seasonings. 5. Cauliflower soup: Cauliflower soup is a comforting and nutritious way to incorporate cauliflower into your diet. Simply sauté some onions and garlic in a pot, add chopped cauliflower, vegetable broth, and your favorite seasonings, and simmer until the cauliflower is tender. Then, blend everything together until smooth and creamy. Incorporating cauliflower into your diet can be a delicious and healthy way to add more vegetables to your meals. Give these creative cauliflower recipes a try and see how easy it is to enjoy the power of cauliflower.

Discover the Amazing Benefits of Eating Kohlrabi: The Superfood You Need in Your Diet

With so many different types of fruits and vegetables out there, it can be hard to know which ones to include in your diet. However, there's one superfood that often gets overlooked but can offer amazing health benefits - kohlrabi. This unique vegetable is part of the cabbage family and is packed full of vitamins, minerals, and antioxidants that can improve your health in numerous ways. From boosting your immune system and helping to prevent cancer to maintaining healthy digestion and improving bone health, kohlrabi should definitely be on your list of must-eat foods. In this article, we'll explore the benefits of eating kohlrabi and provide some tips on how to incorporate it into your diet.

1. What is kohlrabi and why is it a superfood?
Kohlrabi is a lesser-known vegetable that is part of the cabbage family. It has a bulbous shape and a pale green, almost alien-like skin. While it may look unusual, kohlrabi is packed with nutrients that make it a true superfood. One cup of kohlrabi contains only 36 calories and is rich in fiber, vitamin C, potassium, and vitamin B6. It also contains small amounts of other important vitamins and minerals like magnesium, calcium, and iron. Kohlrabi is also a great source of antioxidants, which help to protect the body from damage caused by free radicals. These antioxidants can help to prevent chronic diseases such as heart disease, cancer, and Alzheimer's disease. Additionally, kohlrabi has anti-inflammatory properties that can help to reduce inflammation in the body, which is a major contributor to many chronic diseases. Another benefit of kohlrabi is its ability to aid digestion. The high fiber content in kohlrabi can help to keep the digestive system healthy and regular. This can help to prevent constipation and other digestive problems. In summary, kohlrabi is a highly nutritious vegetable that is low in calories and high in fiber, vitamins, and minerals. Its antioxidant and anti-inflammatory properties make it a true superfood that can help to prevent chronic diseases and promote overall health and well-being. If you have not yet tried kohlrabi, it is definitely worth adding to your diet!

2. The nutritional benefits of kohlrabi
Kohlrabi, a member of the cabbage family, is a superfood that offers a whole range of nutritional benefits. This low-calorie vegetable is packed with essential nutrients such as fiber, vitamins, and minerals. It is a great source of vitamin C, which can help boost your immune system, and vitamin B6, which is essential for healthy brain function. Additionally, kohlrabi contains potassium, which can help regulate blood pressure and reduce the risk of heart disease. The fiber content in kohlrabi can also aid in digestion and help with weight loss by making you feel fuller for longer periods. Moreover, kohlrabi is also rich in antioxidants such as carotenoids and flavonoids, which can help prevent cancer and reduce inflammation in the body. With all these nutritional benefits, kohlrabi is a great addition to any diet, and it's versatile in the kitchen too. You can enjoy it shaved raw in salads, roasted as a side dish, or pureed into soups.

3. How to incorporate kohlrabi into your diet
If you are looking to incorporate kohlrabi into your diet, there are many delicious and easy ways to do so. One simple way to prepare kohlrabi is to peel it and slice it into thin, bite-sized pieces. You can then sprinkle a little salt and pepper on top and enjoy it raw. This is a great way to enjoy the crisp, refreshing taste of kohlrabi without cooking it. Another way to enjoy kohlrabi is to roast it in the oven. You can chop it into small pieces and toss it with a little olive oil, salt, and pepper. Roast it in the oven until it is tender and golden brown. This makes for a delicious and healthy side dish or snack. You can also add kohlrabi

to your salads or use it as a substitute for other vegetables in your recipes. It pairs well with many different flavors, so feel free to experiment and find your favorite way to enjoy this superfood. Overall, incorporating kohlrabi into your diet is a great way to get all of the amazing health benefits it offers while also enjoying its delicious taste.

4. Conclusion.
In conclusion, kohlrabi is an incredibly nutritious vegetable that offers many health benefits. It is packed full of vitamins, minerals, and fiber, making it an excellent choice for anyone looking to improve their overall health and wellbeing. From boosting your immune system to promoting healthy digestion, kohlrabi has a lot to offer. With its mild, sweet flavor, it is also a versatile vegetable that can be used in a variety of dishes. Whether you're eating it raw or cooked, kohlrabi is an excellent addition to any diet. So, next time you're at the grocery store or farmers market, be sure to pick up some kohlrabi and start enjoying all of the amazing benefits this superfood has to offer.

The Incredible Health Benefits of Watercress You Need to Know About!

Watercress is a small, leafy green vegetable that is not as well-known as other members of the Brassicaceae family, like broccoli and kale, but it is just as nutritious, if not more so. In fact, watercress has been hailed as a superfood for centuries, and it has been cultivated for medicinal and culinary purposes since ancient times. This vibrant green leafy vegetable is packed with essential vitamins and minerals, antioxidants, and phytonutrients, which can promote good health and prevent a wide range of diseases. Whether you are looking to improve your digestion, boost your immune system, prevent cancer, or just eat healthier, this post will introduce you to the incredible health benefits of watercress you need to know about!

1. Introduction to watercress and its history
Watercress is a leafy green vegetable that has been enjoyed for its unique flavor and health benefits for centuries. Its scientific name is Nasturtium officinale, and it is a member of the cruciferous family of vegetables, which also includes broccoli, kale, and cauliflower. The origins of watercress can be traced back to ancient Greece and Rome, where it was cultivated for its medicinal properties. In fact, the Greeks and Romans believed that watercress could cure a variety of ailments, including coughs, colds, and even baldness. In the 19th century, watercress was widely cultivated in Europe and America, and it became a popular food for both the rich and the poor. Today, watercress is still a popular vegetable, thanks to its unique flavor and impressive nutritional profile. It is packed with vitamins, minerals, and antioxidants, making it a great addition to any healthy diet. In this article, we will explore the incredible health benefits of watercress and show you why it should be a staple in your diet.

2. Nutritional value of watercress
Watercress is a nutrient-dense green that is packed with vitamins, minerals, and antioxidants. It has a crisp, peppery flavor that makes it a great addition to salads and sandwiches. Some of the key nutrients found in watercress include vitamin C, vitamin K, vitamin A, and calcium. Vitamin C is important for maintaining a healthy immune system, while vitamin K is essential for blood clotting and bone health. Vitamin A is crucial for healthy vision, while calcium is necessary for strong bones and teeth. Watercress is also a good source of antioxidants, including beta-carotene and lutein. These compounds help to protect the body against damage from free radicals, which can cause cell damage and lead to chronic diseases such as cancer and heart disease. Additionally, watercress is a low-calorie food that is high in fiber, which makes it a great choice for those looking to lose weight or maintain a healthy weight. The high fiber content of watercress can also help to lower cholesterol levels and improve digestive health. Overall, watercress is a nutrient-packed green that offers a wide range of health benefits. Whether you add it to your salads, sandwiches, or smoothies, there are many ways to incorporate this superfood into your diet and reap its many health benefits.

3. Health benefits of watercress, including improved digestion, boosted immune system, and cancer prevention
Watercress is a leafy green vegetable that has been used for centuries for its numerous health benefits. One of the most significant health benefits of watercress is improved digestion. Watercress contains a high amount of dietary fiber and sulfur compounds that help stimulate the digestive system and increase bowel movements, preventing constipation and other digestive issues. Additionally, watercress has been

shown to boost immunity due to its high levels of vitamin C and other immune-boosting compounds. These compounds help prevent infection and promote healthy cell growth, making watercress an excellent addition to any diet. Furthermore, studies have shown that watercress may help prevent cancer. Watercress contains compounds called glucosinolates, which have been shown to have anti-cancer properties. These compounds help prevent cancer by inhibiting the growth and spread of cancer cells, and by promoting the death of abnormal cells. Additionally, watercress is a great source of antioxidants, which help fight inflammation, a known risk factor for cancer. In summary, watercress is a nutrient-dense, leafy green vegetable with a wide range of health benefits. It can help improve digestion, boost immunity, and even prevent cancer. Incorporating watercress into your diet is a simple and effective way to improve your overall health and well-being.

4. How to incorporate watercress into your diet
Watercress is a nutrient-rich vegetable that is packed with vitamins and minerals. Incorporating watercress into your diet is a great way to improve your health and wellbeing. There are many ways to incorporate watercress into your diet. One of the easiest ways is to add it to your salads. Watercress has a delicious, peppery taste that can lend a unique flavor to your salads. You can also add watercress to smoothies or juices for an extra nutrient boost. Another great way to incorporate watercress into your diet is by using it as a garnish for soups or stews. Watercress can also be sautéed or stir-fried like spinach, and added to your favorite dishes. You can also use watercress in place of lettuce on your sandwiches and subs. There are endless possibilities when it comes to incorporating watercress into your diet. Not only does it taste great, but it is also incredibly healthy for you. So why not give it a try and see how easy it is to add watercress to your daily diet?

The Incredible Health Benefits of Eating Turnip Greens You Need to Know.

When it comes to healthy eating, most people tend to focus on popular superfoods like kale or spinach. However, there is another leafy green vegetable that is often overlooked in our diets but packs a surprising amount of health benefits: turnip greens. This often-ignored vegetable is actually a nutritional powerhouse, packed with a variety of vitamins and minerals that have been shown to improve overall health and well-being. From protecting your bones and improving your skin to reducing inflammation and promoting healthy digestion, turnip greens are a must-have addition to your diet. Join us as we explore the incredible health benefits of turnip greens and discover why you should add them to your meals today.

1. What are turnip greens?

If you are looking for a superfood that delivers a powerful nutritional punch, then turnip greens are definitely worth considering. Turnip greens are the leafy greens that grow atop the turnip root, and they are packed with vitamins, minerals, and other nutrients that are essential for good health. These greens have a slightly bitter taste and a chewy texture, making them a great addition to soups, stews, and salads. They are also a popular ingredient in Southern cuisine, where they are often cooked with bacon or ham hocks for added flavor. Turnip greens are a good source of vitamin A, vitamin C, vitamin K, and folate. They also contain significant amounts of calcium, iron, and manganese, as well as smaller amounts of potassium and magnesium. Because of their high nutrient content, turnip greens have been linked to a number of health benefits, including better digestion, improved immune function, and a reduced risk of chronic diseases like heart disease and diabetes. Whether you are looking to improve your overall health or simply add more variety to your diet, turnip greens are definitely worth trying.

2. Nutritional profile of turnip greens

Turnip greens, the often-overlooked part of the turnip plant, are packed with valuable nutrients that are essential for maintaining good health. One cup of cooked turnip greens provides over 200% of your daily recommended intake of vitamin K, which is essential for maintaining strong bones and preventing blood clots. Additionally, turnip greens are an excellent source of vitamin A, vitamin C, and folate, which are all essential for maintaining a healthy immune system. Vitamin A is also important for maintaining healthy eyes and skin, while vitamin C is important for the growth and repair of tissues in the body. Folate is important for pregnant women, as it helps to prevent birth defects. Turnip greens are also a great source of calcium, iron, and potassium, which are essential for maintaining healthy blood pressure, strong bones, and preventing anemia. Not to mention, they are low in calories and high in fiber, making them a great choice for weight loss and digestive health. Incorporating turnip greens into your diet is an easy way to increase your intake of vital nutrients and improve your overall health.

3. Health benefits of turnip greens

Turnip greens are a leafy green vegetable that is often overlooked. However, they are packed with essential vitamins and minerals that provide numerous health benefits. One of the main health benefits of turnip greens is that they are an excellent source of vitamin K. Vitamin K plays a crucial role in blood clotting and bone health. Eating turnip greens regularly can help to maintain healthy bones and prevent osteoporosis. Turnip greens are also a great source of vitamin C, which is essential for maintaining a healthy immune system. Vitamin C is also an antioxidant, which means it can protect the body from harmful free radicals that can cause inflammation and damage to cells. In addition to vitamins K and C, turnip greens are also a good source of fiber, which can help to regulate digestion and prevent constipation. They also contain anti-inflammatory compounds that can help to reduce the risk of chronic diseases such as heart disease and cancer. Finally, turnip greens are low in calories and high in nutrients, making them an excellent choice for those looking to lose weight or maintain a healthy weight. They are also easy to prepare and can be added to a variety of dishes, including soups, stews, and salads. Overall, turnip greens are a nutrient-dense vegetable that provides numerous health benefits. By incorporating them into your diet, you can help to improve your overall health and wellbeing.

4. Ways to add turnip greens to your diet.
Adding turnip greens to your diet can provide a wide range of health benefits. They are rich in nutrients such as vitamins A, C, and K, calcium, iron, and antioxidants. But how can you incorporate turnip greens into your daily meals? Here are some simple ways to do it: 1. Add them to salads: Turnip greens are a great addition to any salad. Combine them with other leafy greens, such as spinach and kale, and add your favorite toppings like nuts, seeds, and fruits. 2. Sauté them as a side dish: Sautéed turnip greens make for a delicious and healthy side dish. Simply heat up a little olive oil in a pan, add some garlic, and sauté the greens until they are tender. 3. Make a soup: Turnip greens are a perfect addition to any soup recipe. Add them to your favorite vegetable soup recipe for an extra punch of nutrition. 4. Use them as a sandwich filling: Turnip greens can be used as a tasty and healthy sandwich filling. Simply add them to your favorite bread with some hummus, avocado, and other veggies. By incorporating turnip greens into your daily meals, you can enjoy their incredible health benefits and add variety to your diet.

Why Bok Choy is the Ultimate Superfood You Need to Add to Your Diet!

Bok choy, also known as Chinese cabbage, is a leafy green vegetable that has been a staple in Chinese cuisine for centuries. Recently, it has gained popularity in other parts of the world as a result of its numerous health benefits. This superfood is low in calories, high in fiber, and packed with vitamins and minerals that are essential for overall health and wellness. In this article, we'll dive deeper into the benefits of bok choy, its nutritional value, and how you can easily incorporate it into your diet to reap its many health benefits. Whether you're looking to improve your digestion, boost your immune system or simply add more greens to your plate, bok choy is the ultimate superfood you need to add to your diet today!

1. What is bok choy?
Bok choy, also known as Chinese cabbage, is a leafy green vegetable that is a member of the cruciferous vegetable family. It is popular in Asian cuisine, but has gained popularity in Western cuisine as well due to its many health benefits. Bok choy has wide, dark green leaves and thick white stalks. It is low in calories and high in nutrients, making it an excellent addition to any diet. The vegetable is rich in vitamins A, C, and K, as well as calcium, iron, and potassium. It is also a good source of fiber and antioxidants. Bok choy has a mild, slightly sweet taste and can be eaten raw or cooked. It is versatile and can be added to salads, stir-fries, soups, and other dishes. If you're looking to add more nutrients to your diet, bok choy is an excellent choice.

2. Nutritional value of bok choy
Bok choy is a popular vegetable with a mild, sweet flavor and is an excellent source of vitamins, minerals, and other nutrients. This cruciferous vegetable is low in calories but high in essential nutrients that your body needs to function properly. One cup of bok choy contains only 9 calories but provides you with 63% of your daily recommended intake of vitamin K, 52% of vitamin C, and a good amount of vitamin A, calcium, iron, and fiber. Vitamin K is essential for healthy bones and blood clotting, while vitamin C is vital for a healthy immune system. Bok choy is also rich in antioxidants, which help to protect your cells from damage caused by free radicals. Additionally, the fiber content of bok choy helps to promote healthy digestion and bowel regularity. With all of these essential vitamins and minerals, it's no wonder that bok choy is considered a superfood that should be added to your diet. Whether you enjoy it cooked or raw, bok choy is a delicious and nutritious addition to any meal.

3. Health benefits of bok choy
Bok choy, also known as Chinese cabbage, is a nutritional powerhouse that offers a wide range of health benefits. It is low in calories and high in essential vitamins and minerals, making it an ideal addition to any healthy diet. One of the most significant health benefits of bok choy is its high content of vitamin C. Just one cup of cooked bok choy provides almost 75% of your daily recommended intake of vitamin C. Additionally, bok choy is a good source of vitamin A, vitamin K, and folate. The vitamin A in bok choy can help keep your vision sharp, while the vitamin K can help support healthy bones. Bok choy also contains antioxidants, which can help protect your cells from damage caused by free radicals. Finally, bok choy is an excellent source of fiber, which can help promote healthy digestion and gut health. Incorporating bok choy into your diet is easy – it can be eaten raw in salads, sautéed as a side dish, or added to soups and stews. With its many health benefits, bok choy is a superfood that should not be overlooked!

4. How to incorporate bok choy into your diet

Bok choy is a nutrient-dense superfood that is easy to incorporate into your diet. One of the easiest ways to consume bok choy is by adding it to soups and stir-fries. It has a mild flavor that can complement many different dishes. Another way to incorporate bok choy into your diet is by adding it to salads. The tender leaves and crunchy stems provide a fresh and unique taste to your salads. Additionally, bok choy can be eaten raw as a snack or in a sandwich. You can also use bok choy as a substitute for lettuce in your sandwiches or wraps. If you are a fan of smoothies, bok choy can also be added to your smoothie recipes. This is a great way to get a lot of nutrients from this superfood in one serving. Lastly, bok choy can be steamed and served as a side dish with a little bit of salt and pepper. By incorporating bok choy into your diet in these various ways, you can enjoy its many health benefits and add some variety to your meals.

"Napa Cabbage: The Nutrient-Packed Superfood You Need in Your Diet"

When we think of superfoods, the first things that come to mind are usually kale, blueberries, or acai berries. However, there's another superfood that deserves just as much attention: Napa cabbage. This cruciferous vegetable, also known as Chinese cabbage, is not only delicious but also packed with nutrients that are essential for our health. From vitamins and minerals to antioxidants and fiber, Napa cabbage has it all. In this article, we'll explore the health benefits of Napa cabbage and provide some tasty recipe ideas to help you incorporate this superfood into your diet.

1. What is Napa cabbage?
Napa cabbage, also known as Chinese cabbage, is a popular vegetable that is widely used in Asian cuisine. It originated in the Beijing region of China and has been enjoyed for centuries due to its delicious flavor and numerous health benefits. Napa cabbage has a pale green color and a unique oblong shape with crinkly leaves that are tender and juicy. It has a mild, sweet, and slightly peppery flavor, making it a versatile ingredient in both raw and cooked dishes. Napa cabbage is packed with nutrients and is an excellent source of vitamins C and K, folate, potassium, and dietary fiber. It also contains antioxidants, which help to protect the body against damage from free radicals. This nutrient-dense vegetable is low in calories and carbohydrates, making it an excellent choice for those looking to maintain a healthy diet. Napa cabbage can be eaten raw in salads, added to soups and stews, stir-fried, or even pickled. In recent years, Napa cabbage has gained popularity in Western cuisine due to its unique flavor and versatility in cooking. It's a great alternative to traditional cabbage, and it's easy to find in most grocery stores. Incorporating Napa cabbage into your diet can provide numerous health benefits, making it an excellent addition to any meal.

2. Health benefits of Napa cabbage
Napa cabbage is a nutrient-packed superfood that can provide a multitude of health benefits. One of the most significant benefits of this delicious vegetable is its high vitamin C content. Just one cup of Napa cabbage contains over 45% of your recommended daily intake of vitamin C, which is essential for boosting your immune system and fighting off infections. Additionally, Napa cabbage is rich in vitamin K, which helps regulate blood clotting and promotes bone health. It also contains vitamin B6, which helps maintain healthy brain function and can help reduce the risk of depression. Aside from vitamins, Napa cabbage is also a great source of dietary fiber, which can help keep you feeling full and satisfied after meals, aiding in weight loss efforts. The vegetable is also low in calories, making it a great option for those looking to reduce their calorie intake. Additionally, Napa cabbage contains powerful antioxidants that can help reduce inflammation in the body, which can lead to a reduced risk of chronic diseases such as heart disease and cancer. Overall, adding Napa cabbage to your diet can provide numerous health benefits and help you maintain optimal health. Try incorporating it into your meals today to start reaping the benefits!

3. How to incorporate Napa cabbage into your diet
Incorporating Napa cabbage into your diet is easy and delicious. One of the simplest ways to enjoy Napa cabbage is to simply chop it up and add it to your salads. It is crunchy, refreshing, and adds a lot of nutrients to your salad. You can also use Napa cabbage in stir-fries or soups. It pairs well with many different types of meats and vegetables. Another great way to enjoy Napa cabbage is to use it as a wrap. You can fill it up with your favorite proteins and veggies for a healthy and satisfying meal. You can also

pickle Napa cabbage, which is a popular side dish in many Asian cuisines. Pickling Napa cabbage is easy and requires very few ingredients. Lastly, you can also make coleslaw with Napa cabbage. This is a great way to enjoy the nutritional benefits of Napa cabbage while satisfying your cravings for a classic side dish. Overall, incorporating Napa cabbage into your diet is simple and delicious. With its crunchy texture and mild flavor, it can be used in many different ways to make your meals healthier and more nutritious.

4. Delicious recipe ideas using Napa cabbage.
Napa cabbage is a nutrient-packed superfood that is incredibly versatile and can add a unique twist to any meal. Here are some delicious recipe ideas that showcase the many ways you can use Napa cabbage in your cooking: 1. Napa Cabbage Salad – Combine thinly sliced Napa cabbage, shredded carrots, sliced cucumbers, and sliced radishes in a large bowl. Drizzle with a simple vinaigrette made of olive oil, vinegar, Dijon mustard, and honey. Toss the salad to coat and serve. 2. Napa Cabbage Kimchi – This Korean recipe is a popular way to use Napa cabbage. Mix together garlic, ginger, fish sauce, gochugaru (Korean red pepper flakes), and salt to make a paste. Rub the paste all over the cabbage leaves and let it ferment for a few days. The result is a tangy, spicy, and flavorful dish that can be enjoyed on its own or as a side dish. 3. Napa Cabbage Rolls – These rolls are stuffed with ground pork, rice, and vegetables and are a great way to enjoy Napa cabbage. Blanch the cabbage leaves in boiling water until they are softened. Then, fill each leaf with the pork and rice mixture and roll it up. Place the rolls in a baking dish and bake in the oven until golden brown on top. 4. Napa Cabbage Stir Fry – This is a great way to use up any leftover Napa cabbage in your fridge. Simply stir fry your favorite protein (chicken, beef, tofu, etc.) with some garlic, ginger, and vegetables like bell peppers and onions. Add the Napa cabbage towards the end and cook until it's wilted and tender. Serve over rice or noodles. These are just a few examples of the many ways you can use Napa cabbage in your cooking. Experiment with different flavors and ingredients to find your perfect recipe.

The Incredible Benefits of Adding Arugula to Your Diet: A Comprehensive Guide.

Are you looking for a new addition to your diet that is both healthy and delicious? Look no further than arugula! This leafy green is packed with nutrients and offers a variety of health benefits. From improving digestion and bone health to reducing inflammation and protecting against cancer, arugula is a superfood that should not be overlooked. In this comprehensive guide, we will explore the nutritional value of arugula, the various health benefits it provides, and how to incorporate it into your diet. Whether you are a seasoned health enthusiast or just starting to make healthier choices, read on to discover why arugula should be a staple in your diet.

1. What is arugula and why is it good for you?
Arugula is a leafy green vegetable that is often used in salads and other dishes. It has a distinctive taste that is slightly bitter and peppery, making it a great addition to many different meals. But what makes arugula so good for you? First of all, arugula is low in calories, making it a great choice for anyone who is trying to eat healthily or lose weight. It is also high in vitamins and minerals, including vitamin C, vitamin K, and calcium. These nutrients are essential for maintaining healthy bones, teeth, and skin, as well as boosting your immune system. One of the most significant benefits of arugula is its high antioxidant content. Antioxidants are compounds that help to protect your body from free radicals, which can cause damage to your cells and DNA. Eating a diet that is high in antioxidants can help to reduce your risk of chronic diseases such as cancer, heart disease, and Alzheimer's. Arugula is also a great source of nitrates, which have been shown to help lower blood pressure and improve exercise performance. Additionally, it contains high levels of chlorophyll, which can help to detoxify your body and aid in digestion. Overall, there are many great benefits to adding arugula to your diet. Whether you are looking to improve your overall health, lose weight, or simply enjoy a delicious and nutritious vegetable, arugula is definitely worth incorporating into your meals.

2. Nutritional value of arugula
Arugula, also known as rocket or salad rocket, is a leafy green vegetable that is packed with nutrients. Arugula is low in calories and high in vitamins A and C, making it an excellent choice for anyone looking to improve their overall health. The vegetable is also rich in potassium, calcium, magnesium, and iron, which are essential minerals that help to support various bodily functions. Additionally, arugula is a good source of fiber, which helps to keep the digestive system healthy and functioning correctly. The nutritional value of arugula makes it an excellent choice for anyone looking to boost their immune system, support healthy digestion, or improve their overall health. The vegetable is also rich in antioxidants, which help to protect the body from damage caused by free radicals. Free radicals are unstable molecules that can cause damage to cells and tissues, leading to disease and aging. In summary, adding arugula to your diet can provide a wide range of benefits. With its low calorie count and high nutritional value, it is an excellent choice for anyone looking to improve their health, support healthy digestion, and boost their immune system. So why not try adding some arugula to your next salad or smoothie and start reaping the benefits today?

3. Health benefits of arugula
Arugula is a leafy green vegetable that belongs to the same family as kale and broccoli. It has a peppery taste and is often used in salads and sandwiches. But did you know that this humble vegetable is packed

with nutrition? Here are some of the incredible health benefits of adding arugula to your diet: 1. Arugula is an excellent source of vitamins and minerals. It is high in vitamin K, which is essential for maintaining healthy bones and blood clotting. It also contains vitamin C, vitamin A, calcium, and iron. 2. Arugula is low in calories and high in fiber, making it an excellent choice for weight loss. The fiber in arugula helps to keep you feeling full for longer periods, which can help you to eat less overall. 3. Arugula is also rich in antioxidants, which help to protect your cells from damage caused by free radicals. This can reduce your risk of chronic diseases such as cancer, diabetes, and heart disease. 4. Arugula has anti-inflammatory properties that can help to reduce inflammation in the body. Chronic inflammation is associated with a wide range of health problems, including arthritis, asthma, and inflammatory bowel disease. 5. Arugula is also an excellent source of nitrates, which can help to lower blood pressure and improve overall cardiovascular health. Incorporating arugula into your diet is a simple way to reap all of these incredible health benefits. Whether you add it to your salads or blend it into your smoothies, this vegetable is an easy and delicious way to improve your overall health and wellbeing.

4. How to incorporate arugula into your diet
Arugula is a versatile green that can be added to many dishes. Here are some easy ways to incorporate this nutrient-packed green into your diet: 1. Salads: The most straightforward way to incorporate arugula into your diet is to add it to your salads. Arugula's peppery flavor can add a unique dimension to your salad's taste. 2. Sandwiches and Wraps: You can add arugula to any sandwich or wrap for an extra nutritional boost. It pairs well with meats, cheese, and other vegetables. 3. Pesto: Arugula pesto is a great alternative to traditional basil pesto. It can be used as a spread or a pasta sauce. 4. Smoothies: Arugula can be added to smoothies for an extra nutritional kick. Its mild taste won't overpower the other ingredients. 5. Topping for Pizza: Arugula makes a great topping for pizza. Add it to your pizza after cooking for a fresh taste. 6. Egg Dishes: Arugula can be added to scrambled eggs, omelets, and frittatas. In conclusion, arugula is a nutrient-rich green that is easy to incorporate into your diet. Whether you add it to your salad or your morning smoothie, arugula can provide numerous health benefits that can improve your overall well-being.

Why Green Leaf Lettuce is the Ultimate Superfood for Your Health.

In recent years, the term "superfood" has been used to describe foods that are rich in nutrients and provide numerous health benefits. One of the vegetables that fit this description is green leaf lettuce. This leafy green has long been a staple in salads and sandwiches, but its nutritional value is often overlooked. Green leaf lettuce is not only low in calories, but it is also packed with vitamins, minerals, and antioxidants that can help boost your overall health. In this article, we will explore the many benefits of green leaf lettuce and why it should be a part of your daily diet. From its ability to promote weight loss and improve digestion to its role in reducing inflammation and promoting healthy skin, you will learn why green leaf lettuce is the ultimate superfood for your health.

1. What is green leaf lettuce?
Green leaf lettuce is a type of leafy vegetable that is widely known for its health benefits. It is a member of the lettuce family and is often used as a base for salads or as a sandwich topping. Green leaf lettuce has a mild, sweet flavor and a delicate texture that makes it a popular choice for many people. This type of lettuce is packed with a variety of nutrients that are essential for maintaining good health. It is an excellent source of vitamins A and K, which are important for healthy eyesight and strong bones. Additionally, green leaf lettuce contains high amounts of fiber, which can improve digestion and lower cholesterol levels. It is also rich in antioxidants, which help protect the body from disease and cellular damage. Green leaf lettuce is also a versatile ingredient that can be used in a variety of dishes. It can be eaten raw in salads or used as a topping for sandwiches and burgers. It can also be sautéed or stir-fried with other vegetables for a delicious and healthy side dish. Overall, green leaf lettuce is a superfood that is both delicious and nutritious, making it a great addition to any healthy diet.

2. Nutritional benefits of green leaf lettuce
Green leaf lettuce is one of the healthiest foods you can add to your diet. It is low in calories, high in fiber, and rich in vitamins and minerals. Here are some of the nutritional benefits of green leaf lettuce: 1. Low in calories: A single cup of green leaf lettuce contains only 5 calories. This makes it a great choice for anyone who is trying to lose weight or maintain a healthy weight. 2. High in fiber: Green leaf lettuce is an excellent source of dietary fiber. One cup of lettuce contains 1 gram of fiber, which can help to promote healthy digestion and prevent constipation. 3. Rich in vitamins and minerals: Green leaf lettuce is packed with vitamins and minerals, including vitamin A, vitamin C, vitamin K, iron, and calcium. Vitamin A is essential for healthy vision, while vitamin C is important for a strong immune system. Vitamin K is necessary for healthy bones, and iron and calcium are important for maintaining healthy blood and bones. 4. Antioxidant properties: Green leaf lettuce is rich in antioxidants, which can help to protect your body against damage from harmful free radicals. Antioxidants can also help to reduce the risk of chronic diseases, such as cancer and heart disease. In conclusion, green leaf lettuce is a nutritional powerhouse that can help to promote overall health and wellness. By adding it to your diet, you can reap the many benefits of this ultimate superfood.

3. Health benefits of consuming green leaf lettuce
Green leaf lettuce is one of the healthiest types of vegetables available. It is an excellent source of nutrients, including vitamins A, C, and K, calcium, iron, and fiber. Here are some of the health benefits of consuming green leaf lettuce: 1. Heart health: Green leaf lettuce is low in calories and high in fiber, which can help

reduce the risk of heart disease. The vitamin C and beta-carotene in green leaf lettuce also help to protect the heart by reducing inflammation. 2. Digestive health: The high fiber content in green leaf lettuce can help improve digestion and prevent constipation. It also helps to promote the growth of beneficial gut bacteria, which are important for overall digestive health. 3. Eye health: The vitamin A content in green leaf lettuce is essential for good eye health. It helps to protect the eyes from damage caused by free radicals and can help prevent age-related macular degeneration. 4. Immune system: Green leaf lettuce is a rich source of vitamin C, which is important for a healthy immune system. It helps to boost the production of white blood cells, which fight off infections and diseases. 5. Weight management: Green leaf lettuce is a low-calorie and nutrient-dense food, making it an excellent choice for weight management. It can help keep you full for longer periods, reducing the need for snacking and overeating. In conclusion, consuming green leaf lettuce is an excellent way to provide your body with essential nutrients while supporting overall health and wellbeing. Incorporating it into your diet can lead to a healthier lifestyle and help prevent various diseases and health conditions.

4. How to incorporate green leaf lettuce into your diet
Green leaf lettuce is a superfood that is packed with nutrients and antioxidants that are great for your health. If you're looking for ways to incorporate this leafy vegetable into your diet, there are many options available to you. You can add green leaf lettuce to your sandwiches, wraps, or burgers for a healthy crunch. You can also toss it into your salads for an extra dose of vitamins and minerals. Another great way to enjoy green leaf lettuce is to sauté it with some garlic and olive oil for a quick and easy side dish. You can even add it to your smoothies or juices for a boost of nutrients. If you're looking for a new way to enjoy green leaf lettuce, try using it as a leafy wrap. Simply fill it with your favorite protein, vegetables, and dressing, and you've got a healthy and delicious meal. With so many ways to incorporate green leaf lettuce into your diet, it's easy to see why it's the ultimate superfood for your health.

Chicory Greens: The Nutritious and Delicious Addition to Your Diet.

Are you tired of eating the same old salad greens every day? Do you want to add something new to your diet that is both nutritious and delicious? Look no further than chicory greens! These leafy greens are packed with vitamins and minerals, and their slightly bitter taste adds a unique flavor to any dish. Chicory greens are also incredibly versatile, they can be eaten raw in salads, sautéed as a side dish, or even roasted for a crunchy snack. In this post, we will explore the many health benefits of chicory greens, as well as share some delicious recipes to help you incorporate them into your diet. So, let's get started and discover the wonders of chicory greens!

1. What are chicory greens?

Chicory greens are a type of leafy green vegetable that are often used in salads, soups, and stews. They have a slightly bitter taste, which makes them a great addition to many dishes. Chicory greens come in two main types: curly endive and escarole. Curly endive has curly leaves and is often used in salads, while escarole has broad leaves and is better suited for soups and stews. Chicory greens are also highly nutritious, with a variety of vitamins and minerals. They are rich in vitamin A, which is essential for healthy eyes and skin, and vitamin K, which helps with blood clotting and bone health. Chicory greens also contain calcium, iron, and potassium, important minerals that help keep your body functioning properly. In addition to their nutritional value, chicory greens are also a great low-calorie addition to any diet. They are low in calories and high in fiber, making them a great choice for those looking to lose weight or maintain a healthy weight. Overall, chicory greens are a delicious and nutritious addition to any diet. They add flavor and texture to a variety of dishes and can help keep your body healthy and functioning properly.

2. Health benefits of chicory greens

Chicory greens are a highly nutritious addition to your diet that provide a wide range of health benefits. One of the most significant benefits is their high fiber content, which helps to keep your digestive system healthy and regular. Chicory greens are also an excellent source of vitamins and minerals such as vitamin C, calcium, iron, and potassium. These nutrients play a crucial role in maintaining good health and keeping your body functioning at its best. Additionally, chicory greens are known to have anti-inflammatory properties, which can help to reduce inflammation throughout the body and reduce the risk of chronic diseases such as heart disease, diabetes, and cancer. They also contain antioxidants, which help to protect your body against damage from free radicals. Incorporating chicory greens into your diet is an easy and delicious way to improve your overall health and wellbeing. They can be easily added to salads, smoothies, and other dishes, making them a versatile choice for any meal.

3. How to use chicory greens in your diet

If you're looking to add some greens to your diet, chicory greens are an excellent choice. They are not only nutritious but also delicious. So, how can you use chicory greens in your diet? There are many ways to eat these leafy greens, and the possibilities are endless. One of the simplest ways to use chicory greens is to add them to your salads. They have a slightly bitter taste that pairs well with sweeter fruits like pears or apples. You can also use them as a base for your salad instead of traditional lettuce. When cooked, chicory greens become tender and less bitter, making them a great addition to soups and stews. Another way to use chicory greens is to sauté them and serve them as a side dish. Simply add some garlic, salt, and pepper to a pan and sauté the greens until they are tender. You can also add them to your sandwiches or wraps as a substitute for lettuce. Chicory greens can also be used to make delicious and healthy smoothies. Blend them with your favorite fruits and vegetables for a nutrient-packed drink. They're also a great addition to green juices and can add an extra boost of vitamins and minerals. In conclusion, there are many ways to use chicory greens in your diet. Whether you eat them raw in salads or cooked in soups, they are a versatile and nutritious addition to any meal.

4. Chicory greens recipe ideas.
Chicory greens are a delicious and nutritious addition to any diet, and there are many ways to enjoy them. Here are a few chicory greens recipe ideas to get you started: 1. Chicory and Citrus Salad: Chop up some chicory greens and mix with sliced oranges, grapefruit, and a few slices of red onion. Add a little olive oil and lemon juice to dress. 2. Chicory and Pesto Panini: Spread some pesto on a whole-grain bread slice and layer with cooked chicory greens, roasted red peppers, and sliced mozzarella cheese. Toast it in a panini press. 3. Chicory and White Bean Soup: Sauté some diced onions and garlic in olive oil in a pot, then add chopped chicory greens, canned white beans, and chicken broth. Simmer until the greens are tender and season with salt and pepper. 4. Grilled Chicory Greens: Brush some chicory greens with olive oil and season with salt and pepper. Grill them for a few minutes on each side until they are lightly charred. 5. Chicory and Bacon Quiche: Cook some bacon and crumble it into a pie crust. Whisk together eggs, cream, and chopped chicory greens and pour it over the bacon. Bake until the filling is set. These are just a few chicory greens recipe ideas to inspire you. Get creative and try different combinations of flavors to find your favorite way to enjoy this nutritious and delicious green.

Radish: A Crunchy and Nutritious Delight! Exploring the Health Benefits of Eating Radish.

Radishes are an often-overlooked vegetable that is crunchy, refreshing, and packed with nutrients. This root vegetable is not only delicious but also very healthy. Radishes are low in calories, high in fiber, and loaded with antioxidants, vitamins, minerals, and phytochemicals. They are commonly used in salads, sandwiches, and pickling but they can be enjoyed in so many ways. In this article, we will explore the health benefits of eating radish, including its ability to improve digestion, boost the immune system, fight inflammation, and so much more. Whether you are a fan of this crunchy delight or have never tried it before, read on to discover the many health benefits of adding radish to your diet.

1. What is radish and why is it good for you?
Radishes are a root vegetable that are known for their crunchy texture and peppery flavor. They come in a variety of colors and sizes, ranging from small and round to large and oblong. Radishes are a great source of vitamin C, potassium, and fiber. They also contain antioxidants and other beneficial plant compounds that can help protect against chronic diseases. Eating radishes can help promote healthy digestion, as they contain fiber that can help keep you feeling full and satisfied. They also contain compounds that can help ease inflammation in the body, which can be beneficial for those with conditions such as arthritis. Radishes have also been shown to have antibacterial and antifungal properties, which can help protect against infections. In addition to their health benefits, radishes are a versatile vegetable that can be eaten raw or cooked. They can be sliced thin and added to salads, or roasted and served as a side dish. Radishes can also be pickled for a tangy and flavorful snack. Overall, radishes are a delicious and nutritious vegetable that can be a great addition to any diet. Whether you're looking to boost your intake of vitamins and minerals or simply looking for a new vegetable to add to your meals, radishes are definitely worth trying!

2. Nutritional value of radish
Radish is a root vegetable that is not only delicious but also nutritious. It is low in calories and high in essential nutrients such as vitamin C, folate, and potassium. Consuming radish can help boost your immune system, promote healthy digestion, and reduce the risk of chronic diseases like cancer, heart disease, and diabetes. Radish is also high in dietary fiber, which promotes a healthy digestive system and helps you feel full for longer periods of time. Additionally, radish contains antioxidants that help protect your cells from damage caused by free radicals. These antioxidants have anti-inflammatory properties that help reduce inflammation in the body, leading to a lower risk of chronic diseases. Overall, radish is a great vegetable to include in your diet due to its low-calorie content and high nutritional value. You can enjoy radish in salads, sandwiches, and other dishes, making it easy to incorporate into your daily diet.

3. Health benefits of radish
Radish, a crunchy and nutritious delight, has a plethora of health benefits that are often overlooked. Firstly, radishes are low in calories and high in fiber, making them an excellent choice for those who want to lose weight. They are also a great source of vitamins C, E, and K, which can boost your immune system and help fight infections. In addition, radishes contain antioxidants that can help reduce the risk of chronic diseases like cancer and heart disease. Radishes are also high in potassium, which is essential for maintaining healthy blood pressure levels. The potassium in radishes can help reduce the risk of stroke and heart disease. Moreover, radishes can help improve digestion and relieve constipation due to their

high fiber content. The water content in radishes also helps keep the body hydrated, making them a great food choice during hot weather. In conclusion, radishes are a great addition to any healthy diet. They are low in calories, high in fiber and essential vitamins and minerals, and have many health benefits. Including radishes in your diet can help you maintain a healthy weight, improve your immune system, and reduce the risk of chronic diseases. So, try adding a few slices of radish to your next salad or sandwich and enjoy the health benefits of this crunchy and nutritious delight!

4. How to incorporate radish into your diet
Radishes are a delicious and nutritious vegetable that can be enjoyed in a variety of ways. If you're looking to incorporate more radishes into your diet, here are a few ideas: 1. In Salads: Radishes add a nice crunch and flavor to salads. You can slice them thinly and add them to mixed greens, or chop them up and mix them with other vegetables like cucumber, carrots, and peppers. 2. As a Snack: Radishes make a great snack on their own. Simply wash them, trim the ends, and enjoy them raw. 3. Roasting: Roasting radishes brings out their natural sweetness and makes them a great side dish. You can toss them in olive oil, salt, and pepper, and roast them in the oven until tender. 4. Pickling: Pickling radishes is a great way to preserve them and add flavor. You can make quick-pickled radishes by combining them with vinegar, sugar, salt, and water. 5. Soup: Radishes can be used to flavor soups and stews. You can add them to vegetable soup or make a radish soup by sautéing them with onion and garlic, then simmering them with broth and herbs. Overall, incorporating radishes into your diet is a great way to add variety and nutrition to your meals. With so many ways to enjoy them, you're sure to find a few favorite recipes that include this delicious and nutritious vegetable.

Here Are The Incredible Health Benefits of Eating Basil Every Day.

Basil, also known as the "king of herbs", has been used for thousands of years for its medicinal properties as well as its culinary applications. This herb is not only delicious but also packed with nutrients that can help improve your overall health. From improving digestion and reducing inflammation to protecting against cancer and reducing stress, basil is an herb that should not be ignored. In this article, we will dive into the incredible health benefits of incorporating basil into your daily diet. Whether you add fresh basil to your salads or use it as a garnish on your dishes, you are sure to reap the benefits of this amazing herb. So, keep reading to discover why basil should be a staple in your kitchen for a healthier lifestyle.

1. What is Basil and its Nutritional Value?
Basil is a herb that has been used for centuries in cooking and for medicinal purposes. It is native to Africa and Asia but is now widely grown around the world. Basil has a unique and delicious taste that makes it a favorite herb in many cuisines, especially Italian and Thai dishes. In addition to its culinary uses, basil has many health benefits that make it a valuable addition to any diet. Basil is a nutrient-rich herb that is packed with vitamins and minerals. It is an excellent source of vitamin K, which is essential for blood clotting and bone health. Basil also contains vitamin A, which is important for eye health and immune function. It is also a good source of vitamin C, which is a powerful antioxidant that helps to protect cells from damage caused by free radicals. In addition to its vitamins, basil is also rich in minerals such as calcium, iron, and magnesium. These minerals are essential for maintaining strong bones and teeth, healthy muscles, and proper nerve function. Basil is also a good source of fiber, which helps to promote healthy digestion and can lower cholesterol levels. Overall, basil is a nutritious herb that is low in calories and high in nutrients. It is a great way to add flavor to your meals while also boosting your health.

2. How Basil Can Improve Your Digestion
Basil is a herb that has been used for centuries for its medicinal properties. One of the main benefits of basil is its ability to improve digestion. Basil contains essential oils that have been shown to help relieve bloating, gas, and stomach cramps. It also has anti-inflammatory properties that can help soothe indigestion and heartburn. Basil can stimulate the digestive enzymes that break down food, which can improve your overall digestive health. Additionally, basil can help stimulate the liver and kidneys, which can help remove toxins from the body. It's important to note that basil should be consumed in moderation, as consuming too much can cause digestive issues. A few leaves of basil added to your meals every day can help you improve your digestion, and avoid common digestive issues such as bloating, gas, and indigestion.

3. How Basil Can Help Reduce Inflammation
Basil is not only a flavorful herb but also has incredible health benefits. One of the most notable benefits of eating basil every day is its ability to reduce inflammation. Inflammation is a natural process in the body, but when it becomes chronic, it can lead to various health problems. Basil contains essential oils, including eugenol, citronellol, and linalool, that have anti-inflammatory properties. These oils can help reduce inflammation in the body, which can help prevent chronic diseases such as heart disease, cancer, and arthritis. Additionally, basil also contains flavonoids, which are antioxidants that can help protect the body from free radical damage. Free radicals can cause oxidative stress in the body, leading to inflammation and chronic diseases. By consuming basil every day, you can help reduce inflammation and

oxidative stress in your body, leading to better health and well-being. Basil is a versatile herb and can be added to a variety of dishes, making it easy to incorporate into your daily diet.

4. Other Health Benefits of Basil
Apart from its fabulous taste and aroma, basil has numerous health benefits that you can take advantage of by adding it to your daily diet. One of the most important health benefits of basil is its anti-inflammatory properties. Basil contains essential oils that can help reduce inflammation in the body. This makes it an excellent addition to the diets of people with inflammatory conditions, such as arthritis or asthma. In addition to its anti-inflammatory properties, basil can also help to reduce stress and anxiety. This is because it contains compounds that have a calming effect on the nervous system. Basil is also known to have antibacterial properties. Studies have shown that basil essential oil can help to fight off harmful bacteria, such as E.coli and Salmonella. This makes it an excellent addition to your diet if you are trying to boost your immune system. Finally, basil has been found to be rich in antioxidants, which can help to protect the body from damage caused by free radicals. This can help to prevent cancer, heart disease, and other chronic illnesses. All in all, basil is a great addition to your daily diet, and its health benefits are numerous. So why not try adding some fresh basil leaves to your next meal and enjoy all the benefits it has to offer?

The Secret Benefits of Cilantro: Why You Should Add it to Your Diet Today.

Cilantro, also known as coriander, is a popular herb used in many cuisines around the world. It has a distinct flavor, aroma, and a long list of health benefits that many people are unaware of. Cilantro is an excellent source of vitamins A, C, and K, as well as minerals such as calcium, iron, and potassium. It's also known for its powerful antioxidant and anti-inflammatory properties, which can help to reduce the risk of chronic diseases such as heart disease, cancer, and diabetes. In this article, we will dive into the secret benefits of cilantro and why you should add it to your diet today. Whether you're a seasoned chef or a home cook, this herb is a versatile ingredient that can add flavor, nutrition, and health benefits to your meals.

1. What is cilantro?
Cilantro is a herb that is used in cooking all over the world. It is also known as coriander and is often used as a garnish or in condiments. Cilantro is a member of the parsley family and has a distinctive flavor that is often described as citrusy or slightly sweet. It is commonly used in Mexican, Indian, Middle Eastern, and Asian cuisine. Cilantro is packed with nutrients and has many health benefits. It is rich in vitamins A, C, and K, as well as minerals like calcium, potassium, and iron. Cilantro also contains antioxidants, which can help to protect your body from oxidative stress. Additionally, cilantro has been shown to have antibacterial and antifungal properties, making it a great natural remedy for a variety of ailments. Whether you are looking to improve your health or simply add some flavor to your dishes, cilantro is a great addition to any diet.

2. The nutritional benefits of cilantro
Cilantro, also known as coriander, is a herb that is used in many different cuisines around the world. Not only is it a delicious ingredient, but it also has a lot of nutritional benefits. Cilantro is known to be rich in vitamins A, C, and K, as well as minerals such as calcium, iron, and potassium. These vitamins and minerals help to support a healthy immune system, promote healthy bones, and maintain healthy blood pressure levels. Cilantro is also packed with antioxidants, which help to protect the body from harmful free radicals that can cause damage to cells. Furthermore, cilantro is known to have anti-inflammatory properties, which can help to reduce the risk of chronic diseases such as heart disease and certain types of cancer. Additionally, studies have shown that cilantro can aid in digestion and help to detoxify the body. With all of these nutritional benefits, it's no wonder that cilantro is such a popular ingredient in many different dishes. So, if you're looking to add some extra nutrition to your diet, be sure to add cilantro to your grocery list today!

3. The medicinal benefits of cilantro
Cilantro, also known as coriander, is an herb that is commonly used in cooking. However, many people are unaware of the medicinal benefits of cilantro. This herb is a great source of antioxidants, which are important for fighting diseases. It also has anti-inflammatory properties, which can help reduce the risk of heart disease, arthritis, and other chronic conditions. Cilantro is also known for its ability to help detoxify the body. It can help to remove heavy metals from the body, which can be harmful if they build up over time. Additionally, cilantro has been shown to have antibacterial properties, making it an effective natural remedy for infections. It can also help to improve digestion and reduce bloating. Lastly, cilantro has been shown to have a positive effect on mental health. It can help to reduce anxiety and promote

relaxation. Overall, adding cilantro to your diet can provide many health benefits and is a great way to stay healthy and happy.

4. How to incorporate cilantro into your diet.
If you're interested in adding cilantro to your diet, there are many ways to incorporate this flavorful herb into your meals. One of the simplest ways to enjoy cilantro is to chop it up and sprinkle it over your favorite dishes. It adds a fresh burst of flavor to everything from tacos and salads to soups and stews. You can also blend cilantro into smoothies or juices for a nutrient-packed drink. Cilantro is also a great addition to homemade salsa, guacamole, and hummus. Another great way to incorporate cilantro into your diet is by using it as a garnish for your meals. This is a perfect way to add color and flavor to any dish. Finally, if you're feeling adventurous, you can try cooking with fresh cilantro leaves. Cilantro is a great addition to many dishes, including curries, stir-fries, and marinades. Regardless of how you choose to enjoy cilantro, it's an excellent way to add flavor and nutrition to your diet.

The Power of Parsley: Surprising Health Benefits You Need to Know!

Parsley is a widely known herb that is typically used as a decorative garnish on top of dishes or as a flavoring agent. However, what many people don't realize is that parsley is also packed with numerous health benefits that can make a significant impact on your overall well-being. This green herb is rich in vitamins and minerals that can help fight against various diseases and improve various functions in your body. From reducing inflammation to improving digestion and even protecting against cancer, the benefits of parsley are numerous. In this article, we will explore the surprising health benefits of parsley and how you can incorporate it into your diet to improve your health.

1. Introduction to parsley and its nutritional value

Parsley is a popular herb that has been used for centuries for both culinary and medicinal purposes. It is known for its bright green color, fresh flavor, and versatility in cooking. However, what many people may not know is that parsley also has a surprising amount of nutritional value and health benefits. Parsley is a rich source of vitamins A, C, and K, as well as folate and iron. It is also a good source of antioxidants and other beneficial plant compounds. In this blog post, we'll take a closer look at the nutritional value of parsley and explore the various health benefits associated with its consumption. From reducing inflammation to supporting heart health, parsley is a powerful herb that deserves a place in any healthy diet.

2. Parsley as an anti-inflammatory agent

Parsley is a versatile herb that is commonly used as a garnish or seasoning in many dishes. However, it also has some amazing health benefits that are often overlooked. One of these benefits is its ability to act as an anti-inflammatory agent. Parsley contains a compound known as apigenin, which has been shown to have anti-inflammatory properties. This makes it an excellent herb to use for those suffering from inflammatory conditions such as arthritis, asthma, and even cancer. Additionally, parsley is high in antioxidants, which help to fight inflammation and protect the body from damage caused by free radicals. It is also a good source of vitamins A, C, and K, which are essential for maintaining good health. Incorporating parsley into your diet is easy, as it can be used in a variety of dishes such as salads, soups, stews, and sauces. It can also be enjoyed as a tea or used as a natural remedy for various ailments. Overall, parsley is a powerful herb that should not be underestimated when it comes to its health benefits.

3. Parsley for improved digestion and kidney function

Parsley is a superfood that has many health benefits. One of the most surprising benefits of parsley is its ability to improve digestion and kidney function. Parsley is high in antioxidants, which support the digestive system by reducing inflammation and protecting against damage caused by free radicals. It is also a natural diuretic, which means that it helps to flush toxins out of the kidneys and urinary tract. Parsley contains a compound called apiol that has been known to help reduce the formation of kidney stones. Furthermore, parsley is rich in vitamins and minerals that are essential for healthy digestion, such as fiber and vitamin C. It also contains essential oils that help to stimulate the digestive system, relieving bloating and constipation. So if you're looking for a natural way to improve your digestive health and kidney function, try adding parsley to your diet. You can sprinkle it on top of salads or soups, blend it into smoothies, or use it as a garnish for your favorite dishes.

4. Parsley as a cancer-fighting agent

Parsley is a herb with a lot of health benefits. One of the most surprising health benefits of parsley is its ability to help fight cancer. Parsley contains a variety of compounds that are known for their cancer-fighting properties. One of the most important of these compounds is called apigenin. Apigenin is a flavonoid that has been shown to have potent anti-cancer properties. It has been shown to inhibit the growth of cancer cells and induce apoptosis (cell death) in cancer cells. In addition to apigenin, parsley also contains other compounds that are known to have cancer-fighting properties, including myristicin, limonene, and eugenol. These compounds have been shown to help prevent the formation of cancerous cells and reduce the risk of cancer. So, if you want to take advantage of the cancer-fighting properties of parsley, consider adding it to your diet today!

ABOUT THE AUTHOR

Telesha Cutler is the founder of Profound By Nature and an accredited nutritionist as well as health and wellness coach. To contact author for consultation and diet you may do so by emailing her at teleshacutler@gmail.com.